Access to Health Care Among TRICARE-Covered Children

JOACHIM O. HERO, COURTNEY A. GIDENGIL, NABEEL SHARIQ QURESHI, TERRI TANIELIAN, CARRIE M. FARMER

Prepared for the Defense Health Agency
Approved for public release; distribution unlimited

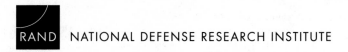

NATIONAL DEFENSE RESEARCH INSTITUTE

For more information on this publication, visit **www.rand.org/t/RRA472-1**.

About RAND

The RAND Corporation is a research organization that develops solutions to public policy challenges to help make communities throughout the world safer and more secure, healthier and more prosperous. RAND is nonprofit, nonpartisan, and committed to the public interest. To learn more about RAND, visit www.rand.org.

Research Integrity

Our mission to help improve policy and decisionmaking through research and analysis is enabled through our core values of quality and objectivity and our unwavering commitment to the highest level of integrity and ethical behavior. To help ensure our research and analysis are rigorous, objective, and nonpartisan, we subject our research publications to a robust and exacting quality-assurance process; avoid both the appearance and reality of financial and other conflicts of interest through staff training, project screening, and a policy of mandatory disclosure; and pursue transparency in our research engagements through our commitment to the open publication of our research findings and recommendations, disclosure of the source of funding of published research, and policies to ensure intellectual independence. For more information, visit www.rand.org/about/principles.

RAND's publications do not necessarily reflect the opinions of its research clients and sponsors.

Published by the RAND Corporation, Santa Monica, Calif.
© 2021 RAND Corporation
RAND® is a registered trademark.

Library of Congress Cataloging-in-Publication Data is available for this publication.

ISBN: 978-1-9774-0632-3

Cover photo: Lesley Atkinson/U.S. Army.

Preface

The nature of military service means that caregivers of children from military families—especially children with complex health care conditions—may have more difficulty than caregivers of civilian children when it comes to accessing and coordinating health care. The Military Health System has made numerous policy changes over the past decade to improve access to care for all beneficiaries, but the implications of these changes for military families is not well understood. A recent analysis of data from the national Medical Expenditure Panel Survey found that self-reported access to routine and specialty care for TRICARE-covered children was lower than for children in other coverage categories, raising questions within the U.S. Department of Defense and among the public. To gain a clearer picture of military families' health care experiences and ability to access needed health care, the Defense Health Agency asked the RAND Corporation to investigate the adequacy of access to pediatric care for TRICARE-covered children.

This report presents the findings and recommendations from an analysis of data from the National Survey of Children's Health, which is a large, nationally representative survey sponsored by the Health Services and Resources Administration of the U.S. Department of Health and Human Services, as well as an analysis of data from a survey sponsored by Blue Star Families, a military service organization. The results and recommendations should be of interest to policymakers, service members and their families, and organizations that support military families.

The research reported here was completed in October 2020 and underwent security review with the sponsor and the Defense Office of Prepublication and Security Review before public release.

This research was sponsored by the Defense Health Agency and conducted within the Forces and Resources Policy Center of the RAND National Security Research Division (NSRD), which operates the National Defense Research Institute (NDRI), a federally funded research and development center sponsored by the Office of the Secretary of Defense, the Joint Staff, the Unified Combatant Commands, the Navy, the Marine Corps, the defense agencies, and the defense intelligence enterprise.

For more information on the RAND Forces and Resources Policy Center, see www.rand.org/nsrd/frp or contact the director (contact information is provided on the webpage).

Contents

Figure and Tables

Figure

Tables

Summary

Military children often face unique stressors that can affect their health care needs and the level of care they receive, including frequent moves, limited pediatric provider options when parents are posted to geographically remote installations, the stresses of deployment, and limited informal support networks to help with special health care needs (SHCN).

TRICARE, the U.S. Department of Defense (DoD) insurance program for eligible service members and their dependents, provides health care coverage to nearly 2 million children under the age of 18 (Defense Health Agency, 2020). These children receive health care either at on-base military treatment facilities (MTFs) or from a network of contracted providers. Prior DoD evaluations have found that TRICARE meets internal standards for access for child beneficiaries (Defense Health Board, 2017; Office of the Secretary of Defense, 2014), but survey results suggest that TRICARE-covered children may have less access to care than children with other sources of insurance and, in some cases, children with no insurance coverage. In response to these findings, DoD asked the RAND Corporation to investigate potential gaps and to identify opportunities to improve health care for military children.

Measures of Health Care Access and Quality for TRICARE-Covered Children

Two DoD surveys monitor TRICARE beneficiaries' experiences with pediatric providers: the Joint Outpatient Experience Survey (JOES), which includes separate surveys for patients who receive care at MTFs and from contracted providers in the TRICARE network, and the Health Care Survey of DoD Beneficiaries (HCSDB), which solicits feedback from adult TRICARE beneficiaries on access to care in a way that allows comparison with other insurance programs.[1] However, the HCSDB has not included questions about pediatric care experiences since 2010 and the JOES does not collect data on children older than age 10. The Military Health System Data Repository contains information on pediatric health care utilization and quality but does not capture comprehensive data on patient experiences.

To address these data-collection gaps, we analyzed alternative sources of data on access to services for TRICARE-covered children under age 18, including the National Survey of Children's Health (NSCH), which collects data on the physical and emotional health of U.S. children from birth to age 17 (U.S. Census Bureau, undated), and the annual Military Family Lifestyle Survey (MFLS) for 2018, conducted by the nonprofit military family support organization Blue Star Families (undated). We found that the NSCH sample of TRICARE-covered children, as reported by their caregivers, closely matched official DoD data on the sociodemographic characteristics of these children. The MFLS collected data from families via an internet convenience sample and therefore is likely not representative of TRICARE-covered children overall; however, the survey still provides some indication of specific areas of satisfaction and concern for some caregivers of TRICARE-covered children.

We captured perceptions regarding access and quality of care among caregivers of TRICARE-covered children. When possible, we used these measures to compare the experiences of TRICARE-

---

[1]   A third survey, the TRICARE Inpatient Satisfaction Survey, collects patient experience data on hospital stays but does not include pediatric populations.

covered children with those of children who had private insurance, public insurance (through Medicaid or another government assistance program), and no insurance. Among TRICARE-covered children, we also explored differences by duty status, service branch, and specific type of TRICARE coverage (e.g., TRICARE Prime, TRICARE Select) to determine whether these differences were associated with differences in caregivers' perceptions regarding pediatric care access.

Specifically, we used the NSCH data to evaluate pediatric health care access across six domains: usual source of care, specialist care, getting needed care, care coordination, insurance coverage and affordability, and patient-centeredness. Using MFLS data, we examined reported timeliness in seeing a medical provider and obtaining a referral, as well as overall satisfaction with access to care and provider quality.

Key Findings

TRICARE beneficiaries can be enrolled in one of several types of TRICARE plans, depending on eligibility and location. Generally, dependents of service members can be enrolled in either an HMO-type plan known as TRICARE Prime or a PPO-type plan known as TRICARE Select. The primary difference is that dependents enrolled in TRICARE Prime have lower cost-sharing than those in TRICARE Select, but they require a referral for specialty care, and these visits typically need to occur at an MTF. TRICARE Select beneficiaries have higher cost-sharing but more flexibility in providers and do not need referrals to see specialists.

Between 2016 and 2018, caregivers of TRICARE-covered children reported approximately the same level of access to health care as caregivers of children covered by other types of insurance. Both groups reported higher levels of access than uninsured children.

Caregivers of children with any kind of insurance generally reported that coverage was adequate and that providers were responsive to their children's needs. TRICARE-covered children were more likely than commercially insured children to have coverage for mental and behavioral health that met their needs. Their caregivers also reported fewer problems paying for health care (likely due to the lower cost-sharing in TRICARE plans relative to most other insurance) and had greater access to—and need for—care coordination services. However, caregivers of TRICARE-covered and publicly insured children reported more frustration obtaining necessary services than caregivers of commercially insured children.

Compared with children with other types of insurance, TRICARE-covered children were less likely to come from low-income families but relocated more often and were therefore less likely to have a single primary health care provider. They were also more likely to require referrals for various types of specialty care and faced greater difficulty obtaining these referrals.

Access challenges according to several measures were more pronounced for TRICARE-covered children with more-complex health needs. Caregivers of TRICARE-covered children with SHCN had more difficulty getting referrals, were more likely to report that their children did not get needed care, had more frustration getting care, and had a greater desire for more help coordinating care compared with caregivers of TRICARE-covered children without SHCN. However, access experiences were similar among TRICARE-coverage children with SHCN and children with SHCN in other coverage groups.

Service-related relocations among the TRICARE population presented additional challenges for pediatric access. TRICARE-covered children whose families frequently moved reported significantly higher degrees of forgone care, difficulty getting a referral, frustration getting needed services, and a desire for more care coordination than those who had never moved over a child's life.

Among children with TRICARE coverage, those from active-duty families were less likely than children from non–active-duty families to have difficulty obtaining health care (including mental and behavioral health care), and their families were less likely to report trouble paying medical bills. Active-duty families were also less likely to report not getting needed care or having trouble paying health care bills. Caregivers of children with TRICARE Prime with a network primary care manager and those with TRICARE Select were the most likely to agree that these children received timely pediatric care when it was needed and were more satisfied with the overall ease of access and timeliness of their children's health care. These rates were lower for Air Force children, however. Their caregivers also reported greater difficulty obtaining timely referrals and were less satisfied with the quality of providers.

Recommendations

Our findings point to several opportunities for DoD to improve how it tracks and addresses potential gaps in access to care for pediatric TRICARE beneficiaries.

Routinely Collect Pediatric Patient Experience Data

Currently, external data are the only means of comprehensively tracking the health care experiences of the entire population of TRICARE-covered children and assessing those experiences against civilian benchmarks. Legislative changes have made it easier for DoD to collect these data internally, but there is still a need to establish procedures for routine, timely, standardized data collection—such as by resuming fielding of the pediatric survey component of the HCSDB—and to make these data available in a way that facilitates comparison.

Further Streamline Referrals and Monitor Effects on Patient Experiences

Our analysis indicated that the referral process was a source of difficulty for pediatric TRICARE beneficiaries compared with those who had private or public insurance—particularly for children with SHCN. Changes have been underway to streamline and expedite referrals within the Military Health System, but the effects were not yet evident in the data at the time of this research. Going forward, DoD should monitor wait times for referrals and specialty appointments and evaluate the reasons for disparities.

Fully Implement DoD Plans to Monitor the Effects of Permanent Changes of Station and Other Service-Related Relocations

Frequent relocations may exacerbate the challenges that military families face when navigating children's health care options. In response to recent legislation, DoD began monitoring the effects of relocations on children with SHCN. Patient experience data among recently relocated families, combined with administrative data, could be used to determine the effectiveness of programs to mitigate negative effects.

Review the Availability and Use of Care Coordination Services for Children with Complex Health Conditions

Caregivers of TRICARE-covered children with SHCN were more likely than caregivers of other insured children with SHCN to receive care coordination assistance but still reported shortfalls. TRICARE beneficiaries with complex health conditions may be eligible for case management services at no cost. Additionally, primary care managers and 24-hour helplines through Military OneSource and the TRICARE Nurse Advice Line may fulfill limited coordination and assistance roles (TRICARE, 2019). However, our results suggest that a significant degree of demand for such assistance remained unmet in 2016–2018, and administrative data on the use of these services were incomplete. Better access to more-effective care coordination for TRICARE-covered children with SHCN might improve experiences where they lagged behind those of other insurance groups, including difficulty with the referral process and frustration in obtaining needed services. This highlights the need for a broad review of the availability and use of care coordination for children with SHCN to help identify how their needs can be met.

Acknowledgments

We are grateful for the support of our project sponsor, CAPT Edward Simmer, along with Krystyna Bienia at the Defense Health Agency. We greatly appreciate Blue Star Families for sharing their survey data and would like to thank Hisako Sonethavilay and Jessica Strong for their assistance. We are also grateful for the support we received from Rachel Linsner and other staff at the Institute for Veterans and Military Families at Syracuse University. We also thank Jeanne Ringel and Roopa Seshadri for serving as technical peer reviewers; their comments greatly enhanced the quality of the report. Finally, we thank Lauren Skrabala for editorial assistance and Aaron Lang for project and administrative support.

Abbreviations

CAHPS	Consumer Assessment of Healthcare Providers and Systems
DHA	Defense Health Agency
DHB	Defense Health Board
DoD	U.S. Department of Defense
EFMP	Exceptional Family Member Program
FY	fiscal year
GAO	U.S. Government Accountability Office
HCSDB	Health Care Survey of DoD Beneficiaries
HMO	health maintenance organization
ICD	International Classification of Diseases
JOES	Joint Outpatient Experience Survey
MBHCN	mental or behavioral health care needs
MEPS	Medical Expenditure Panel Survey
MFLS	Military Family Lifestyle Survey
MHS	Military Health System
MTF	military treatment facility

NDAA	National Defense Authorization Act
NSCH	National Survey of Children's Health
PCM	primary care manager
PCS	permanent change of station
PPO	preferred provider organization
SHCN	special health care needs

CHAPTER ONE

Introduction

The U.S. Department of Defense (DoD) provides health care coverage to nearly 2 million children under the age of 18 (Defense Health Agency [DHA], 2020). These children, who are enrolled as beneficiaries in DoD's TRICARE program, receive care both at military treatment facilities (MTFs) located on military installations and from a network of providers who are contracted by one of TRICARE's managed care support contractors. Dependents of active-duty, retired, and reserve-component service members can enroll in variants of two basic coverage options, TRICARE Prime and TRICARE Select. TRICARE Prime operates like a staff-model HMO with lower cost-sharing but more restrictions on where and from whom enrollees can receive care. Most care for Prime enrollees must be provided by MTFs, and most kinds of specialty care and care received outside of MTFs require prior authorization and a referral from a primary care manager. TRICARE Select is a PPO option with more cost-sharing but fewer network restrictions and no need for a referral to receive care from covered providers. In fiscal year (FY) 2018, 66 percent of eligible children under age 18 were enrolled in TRICARE Prime, and 32 percent were enrolled in TRICARE Select (DHA, 2019).

Children covered by TRICARE often face circumstances that pose health care access challenges that differ from those of children with other types of health coverage. Frequent moves due to the nature of military service can cause disruptions in routine provider relationships and make it difficult to establish a regular source of care (Gleason and Beck, 2017; U.S. General Accounting Office, 2001).

The stresses of deployment and limited extended family support can restrict families' flexibility to manage care for dependents with special health care needs (SHCN) (Paley, Lester, and Mogil, 2013). Military installations are often located in regions of the country with sparse provider networks, which can limit accessible options, particularly for specialty care. Provider network challenges can be exacerbated for pediatric subspecialties, which are in shorter supply across the U.S. health care system compared with adult specialties (Children's Hospital Association, 2012; Mayer, 2006; Wong et al., 2017).

In acknowledgement of these challenges, DoD has periodically evaluated access to care among children covered by TRICARE, finding that it generally meets the access standards outlined in TRICARE regulations (Defense Health Board [DHB], 2017; Office of the Secretary of Defense, 2014). However, a 2017 DHB report found a divergence between analyses using objective performance measures, which have generally found adequate access, and the testimonials of many military families who struggle to manage care for children with complex health needs (DHB, 2017). A more recent study using public data from the Medical Expenditure Panel Survey (MEPS) suggested that families of children covered by TRICARE may have worse access experiences than families covered by other sources of health care coverage (Seshadri et al., 2019).

Other concerns have been raised by researchers, military service organizations, and other stakeholders regarding access to pediatric care among TRICARE families, including network inadequacy, particularly for specialty care (National Institutes of Health, 2014); travel times (Brown et al., 2015); and frequent need for prior authorization and referrals to receive specialty care (Blue Star Families, 2020).

Over the past decade, the Military Health System (MHS) has implemented numerous policy changes aimed at improving access, including expanding access to mental health providers and services, preventive care, and urgent care (DHA, 2019). It has also relaxed requirements for prior authorization or a referral for some types of care and in some coverage categories (DHA, 2019). In the meantime, the MHS has undergone large administrative changes, including a reduction in the number of administrative regions from three to two and the concentration of management responsibility for MTFs under DHA. Previously, management of these facilities was divided among the Army, Navy, and Air Force. The type of TRICARE coverage that families can enroll in could also mean very different experiences in accessing care.

To better understand these issues and possible variation among TRICARE-covered families, DHA asked the RAND Corporation to explore the challenges that caregivers face in accessing care for their TRICARE-covered children and to identify opportunities to improve health care for these children and their families.

Defining and Measuring Access to Health Care

Access to care is a complex, multifaceted concept, incorporating both structural components of the health care system (such as whether there are enough health care providers) and patients' experience with receiving health care (such as whether patients are able to receive care from providers they are comfortable with). Access to health care is often conceptualized and measured across five domains, sometimes known as the "5 As of access" (Penchansky and Thomas, 1981):

- availability (adequate supply of providers)
- accessibility (distance to care and timeliness)
- accommodation (convenience of care)
- acceptability (patient comfort with providers)
- affordability (nonprohibitive cost).

Some domains of access can be measured through objective assessments. TRICARE regulations (32 CFR 199.17) define access standards for its civilian provider network using objective indicators related to *availability* and *accessibility*. For example, the regulations dictate that provider networks include a "sufficient number and mix of board-certified specialists to meet reasonably the anticipated needs of enrollees." Adequacy of *availability* is evaluated by each of the TRICARE regional offices and reported in network adequacy reports.

Network *accessibility* for TRICARE Prime enrollees is determined by the following standards (32 CFR 199.17):

- Distance: Primary care is available within a 30-minute travel time from a Prime enrollee's home, 60 minutes for specialty care.
- Timeliness: Wait times should be no longer than four weeks for a well-patient visit or specialty care referral, no longer than one week for routine care, and no longer than 24 hours for urgent care appointments. Emergency services should be available 24 hours a day, seven days a week, and in-office wait times for nonemergency visits should not exceed 30 minutes.

In addition to structural factors, such as provider availability, access can be assessed through the lens of patients' experience with care. Along with population health and per capita cost, patient experience of care is one of three dimensions pursued in the Institute of Health Improvement's Triple Aim—reflected in the MHS Quadruple Aim—a framework developed to optimize health system performance (Institute for Healthcare Improvement, undated). Patient experiences are downstream outcomes that are affected by a system's performance in all five domains of access. A widely recognized standard for measuring such experiences is the Consumer Assessment of Healthcare Providers and Systems (CAHPS) set of surveys, which produce standardized measures of access and quality that can be compared across providers and health plans. Such surveys collect information on a variety of topics, such as ease of getting needed care; timely access to routine, specialty, or urgent care; usual source of care, such as a personal health care provider; access to specialized services and family-centered care (including shared decisionmaking); and coordination of care and services (Agency for Healthcare Research and Quality, 2020, 2008).

Measures of Access to Care in the Military Health System
DHA tracks and stores many indicators of pediatric access in the MHS Data Repository. These data are commonly used to assess health care utilization, access, and quality for service members and their families. For example, DHA uses the data to monitor and report on MTF

appointment availability, time between referral and receipt of care, and utilization of different types of care across beneficiary groups. Data on MTF access and quality are publicly available through the MHS Transparency Wizard (MHS, various dates). The data are unavailable for care received through the TRICARE network, however, and there are no publicly available measures of access to pediatric care.

Despite the vast amount of information in the MHS Data Repository, it does not contain comprehensive data on patients' care experiences. Such data on pediatric care are instead collected through two survey tools: the Joint Outpatient Experience Survey (JOES) and the Health Care Survey of DoD Beneficiaries (HCSDB):[1]

- JOES collects information about patients' experiences with outpatient care at MTFs. Patients who receive care through the TRICARE network but not at an MTF complete the clinician and group CAHPS survey, referred to as JOES-C. Both JOES and JOES-C collect information about respondents' experiences with a single health care visit—for example, whether respondents were able to schedule an appointment as soon as they wanted, how well they felt the provider communicated with them during the visit, and their experience with the office staff. JOES surveys are sent to adult patients and caregivers of children from birth to age 10, with an estimated response rate of 8 percent (DHB, 2017). Patient experience is not assessed for pediatric visits for children and adolescents ages 11–17 due to concerns about adolescent health care privacy (DHA, 2020).
- The HCSDB is a large survey of adult TRICARE beneficiaries that collects information on beneficiaries' experiences with TRICARE over the previous 12 months, including perceptions of how easy it was to access care, satisfaction with health care services, and opinions about their health coverage (TRICARE, 2009). Questions about access to care and other aspects of patient experience are closely modeled on the CAHPS survey to allow

---

[1] A third survey, the TRICARE Inpatient Satisfaction Survey, collects patient experience data on hospital stays but does not include pediatric populations.

comparisons between TRICARE and other insurers. DoD used to field a version of the HCSDB that asked caregivers about the care provided to their children younger than 18, but it has not been fielded since 2010.

Prior Assessments of Access to Care for TRICARE-Covered Children

In recent years, there have been several assessments of access to care for children covered by TRICARE. Here, we provide a brief overview of the findings from assessments of pediatric access to MHS care between 2014 and 2019:

- a congressionally mandated study of health care and related support provided to dependent children of members of the armed forces in July 2014 (Office of the Secretary of Defense, 2014)
- an independent review of pediatric health care services by the DHB in December 2017 (DHB, 2017)
- a report to Congress on plans to improve MHS pediatric care and related services in December 2018 (DoD, 2018b)
- research analysis of MEPS data published in the August 2019 issue of the journal *Health Affairs* (Seshadri et al., 2019).

We also reviewed annual TRICARE program reports to Congress that included various metrics related to pediatric services.

Congressionally Mandated Study of Health Care and Related Support for Children of Members of the Armed Forces, July 2014

Section 735 of the National Defense Authorization Act (NDAA) for FY 2013 required the Secretary of Defense to comprehensively assess policies and programs related to the provision of health care and other support to children of members of the armed forces (Pub. L. 112-239, 2013). The study included an assessment of policies regarding pediatric care, access to pediatric and specialty health care for dependents, and adequacy of services for children with SHCN, as well as strategies for mitigating the impact of frequent relocations on health care continuity for children (Office of the Secretary of Defense, 2014). The report concluded that TRICARE and the military departments provided adequate access to high-quality care, including specialty care; however, these conclusions were based on limited and often indirect data. Metrics used in the evaluations included the percentage of care delivered in network, emergency department utilization, and a review of TRICARE regional office network adequacy reports. It is important to note that the study did not analyze targeted metrics that would have enabled an evaluation of pediatric access according to the adequacy standards in the TRICARE manual, such as those related to wait times, referrals, and availability of providers. Data on member experiences related to pediatric care were also not evaluated, but the report did recommend that future evaluations include these more-targeted metrics. Thus, the findings may not have included a sufficiently robust assessment to detect problems.

The study evaluated findings regarding access to routine and specialty care. In each instance, the lead metric for evaluation was the proportion of care delivered in non-network settings. Low levels of non-network care were considered evidence of network adequacy. The study found that 7.2 percent of pediatric care overall, 7 percent of inpatient hospitalizations, 13 percent of same-day surgeries, and 35 percent of emergency department visits were non-network. Rates of non-network care were found to be significantly lower among chronic and specialty-dependent pediatric beneficiaries, defined as beneficiaries with more than two visits to a specialty provider in a year, than among beneficiaries with only a single specialty encounter in a year.

The study also found that network adequacy reports generated by TRICARE regional offices were insufficient to determine the adequacy of care, given that provider lists indicated only whether a provider was in-network, not whether the provider was accepting new patients. The regional office reports also lacked data on individual pediatric specialty providers, preventing an assessment of access to different kinds of specialty care.

Finally, the study evaluated programs to help mitigate disruptions to care from relocations. It found that transfers could result in extended wait times for appointments with specialty providers for children with SHCN. The report recommended a comprehensive system for evaluating care coordination for these children and noted that there was no mechanism for identifying families who were eligible for—not enrolled in—the military's Exceptional Family Member Program (EFMP), which provides support and resources to the families of children with SHCN. Among other resources, EFMP provides coordination benefits and supports that can help families during these transitions.

Despite the conclusions about adequacy of care, significant data restrictions prevented the study team from evaluating adequacy according to the criteria in the TRICARE manual. Instead, the study team used metrics with significant limitations. For instance, the extent to which children may have gone without needed care is not detectible when looking only at encounters that occurred. Additionally, low rates of non-network care, an important metric by which the study team measured adequacy, could just as well reflect high barriers to accessing non-network care as low barriers to accessing in-network care. For most TRICARE beneficiaries at the time, receiving non-network care required an authorization and a referral, and members who could not obtain an authorization would be required to seek care in the network or at an MTF. Therefore, although some care may have been ultimately obtained in network or at an MTF, it may not have been the beneficiary's preferred care.

Review of Pediatric Health Care Services by the Defense Health Board, December 2017

In December 2017, the DHB released a report in response to a request from the Assistant Secretary of Defense for Health Affairs to "examine opportunities to improve the overall provision of health care and related services for children of members of the Armed Forces" (DHB, 2017, p. 32). In carrying out its independent review, the DHB explored several topics, including whether children had ready access to primary and specialty pediatric care, the impact of relocation on children with special mental or behavioral health care needs (MBHCN), access to behavioral health services, and the effects of data limitations on improvement efforts. The report was conducted after the passage of the

NDAA for FY 2017, which included several large structural changes to the MHS and provisions related to pediatric care. The study consisted of a literature review, consultation with subject-matter experts, and analysis of access, satisfaction, and quality data. Importantly, the DHB was able to analyze several metrics that were either unavailable or not considered in the congressionally mandated July 2014 report on pediatric care access (Office of the Secretary of Defense, 2014). Although the independent review concluded that access adequacy standards were generally met, according to available metrics, it found that data were insufficient to evaluate pediatric access effectively. Specifically, the report concluded that the MHS lacked an appropriate focus on patient and family experiences and recommended improvements in data collection, data standardization, and care coordination.

For routine appointments in direct care settings (MTFs), the DHB concluded that pediatric access as measured by time to appointment generally met TRICARE adequacy standards for both acute and nonacute appointments for age groups under 13 years old but fell short of those standards for older age groups. It found that adequacy in meeting access standards varied by MTF, with 33 percent of MTFs falling short of TRICARE standards. As noted, adequacy by this metric was evaluated only for care delivered in an MTF. The study also found that 7 percent of the MHS pediatric population lived in zip codes with a shortage of primary care health professionals, and approximately 30 percent lived in areas with a shortage of mental health professionals. (This data point was especially concerning, given that more than 90 percent of mental health visits were purchased care.) Looking at the rate of preventable admissions, an indirect measure of access to outpatient care, the percentage ranged from 3.7 percent among 13- to 17-year-olds to 11.9 percent among 5- to 8-year-olds in the MHS.

The DHB also found that pediatric specialty care appointments in direct care settings were well within TRICARE adequacy standards, with the average time to appointment at one to two days relative to a 28-day standard of adequacy. However, although the report estimated the number of children with complex health care needs in the MHS using the pediatric medical complexity algorithm, it did not report access to care metrics by complexity.

The DHB report included patient experience data from the JOES and noted differences by branch of service; however, it did not present a benchmark of adequacy or point of comparison. The report concluded that JOES data were insufficient measures of patient experience due to the survey's low response rate, the fact that it was restricted to children age 10 or younger, and its limitation to patient encounters. The DHB noted that it had received numerous public comments regarding difficulties that families faced when accessing pediatric specialty care. However, there was no mention of how these comments were solicited, how many responses were received, or whether the commenters were representative of the beneficiary population. The report simply stated that the DHB had "received numerous public comments that voiced the challenges of navigating the MHS with a child with complex needs, securing referrals, and reestablishing care after a PCS [permanent change of station]" (DHB, 2017, p. 6).

The DHB report noted that new data would be made available to better evaluate time to appointment in direct care and TRICARE network settings, including the time between consult and booking and between booking and appointment. Prior metrics were flawed in that they captured time from booking to appointment only, when TRICARE network referrals might require days from the consult to when an appointment is booked.

Finally, the study looked at the impact of PCS and other service-related relocations on access to care. The report noted that transferring medical records in these cases was solely the responsibility of beneficiaries—service members and their families—unless they were enrolled in the EFMP. It concluded that the MHS did not have optimal care coordination for this purpose and urged uniformity in the handoff during relocation.

Plan to Improve MHS Pediatric Care and Related Services, 2018
Section 733 of the NDAA for FY 2018 required the Secretary of Defense to develop plans to improve pediatric care for the children of service members (Pub. L. 115-91, 2017). The Secretary of Defense

submitted the final report on these plans in December 2018 (DoD, 2018b). That report indicated that DoD planned to develop measures to evaluate access and care coordination, improve data collection and use, increase access to behavioral care, and mitigate the impact of PCS and other relocations on care continuity.

According to the report, the MHS has been developing a centralized pediatric data display for a variety of metrics relating to pediatric care quality and access to address a previously identified need for data on pediatric care. Among the access metrics considered for inclusion were those related to receipt of recommended well-child and preventive care, time-based metrics of access (including referrals, specialty care, and third-next-available appointment), and existing patient experience measures (JOES). The pediatric data display was scheduled to launch by the end of 2019. Similar efforts are in place for behavioral health metrics, on which the DoD Behavioral Health Clinical Community program has begun an annual evaluation of behavioral health care access and utilization. Additional data collection and monitoring efforts are underway to minimize problems with continuity of care for families that relocate, especially for those with complex medical or behavioral needs. The MHS is setting up a centralized approach to tracking metrics, including transferring data between regions, adding warm handoffs when there is a move, and standardizing processes.[2] To support these efforts, the MHS will adopt the GENESIS electronic health record system, which will standardize the collection of access and quality metrics over time.

Together, these efforts should provide significant new means of tracking pediatric care; however, current efforts do not appear to address the need for systemwide measures of patient experience as recommended by the DHB.

---

[2] A *warm handoff* in the MHS is when a family's current and new providers and case workers coordinate with the family and each other to facilitate a smooth transfer of the family's care and services to a new location.

Analysis of Medical Expenditure Panel Survey in the Journal *Health Affairs*, 2019

In 2019, researchers from the Children's Hospital of Philadelphia published a study that used publicly available MEPS data to investigate perceptions of access among TRICARE-covered families relative to families in civilian coverage groups (Seshadri et al., 2019). The MEPS is a set of large-scale surveys on health conditions, health status, health service use, satisfaction with care, and insurance coverage from a nationally representative sample of individuals, families, medical providers, and employers. The researchers used data pooled from multiple years (2007–2015) for households with children under age 17 to examine responses to questions from CAHPS instruments designed to assess various aspects of patient experience.

The study found that TRICARE underperformed relative to other insurance types in two of seven outcomes they investigated, including "accessible care" and "responsive care."[3] Accessible care was a composite that essentially measured ease of access to after-hours care, and responsive care was a composite of whether the providers asked about other treatments received and whether they involved the respondent in the decision process. We note that these categories represent narrow measurements of broad and inconsistently defined concepts. For instance, accessibility often encompasses not only whether the source of care can be easily reached after hours but also whether appointments can be easily scheduled, the timeliness of care, and provider proximity.

The authors compared responses to the survey items based on the respondent's insurance group. In the study, children who were covered by TRICARE were compared with those covered by Medicaid, the Children's Health Insurance Program, and other public insurance; commercial insurance; and no insurance. It also assessed responses for children with complex health care needs (based on the Children with Special Health Care Needs Screener) and for children with a caregiver-

---

[3] We note, however, that the odds-ratio presentation of these results may amplify the significance of these findings. In an appendix to their article, the authors present predicted probabilities in which the only meaningful differences in response are between TRICARE and commercial insurance for the "accessible" and "responsive" care questions.

reported behavioral health diagnosis. The authors noted several limitations to their analysis, including biases inherent to self-reported data, small sample sizes (and thus large standard errors), and timing challenges between reporting on insurance coverage and perceptions of health care quality.

Summary of Prior Assessments

Evaluations of TRICARE-covered children's access to care conducted in the past five years have relied on differing metrics to evaluate the adequacy of pediatric access. Despite these differences, these prior studies determined that available objective metrics generally indicate adequate levels of access for TRICARE-covered children. For example, the 2014 report to Congress (Office of the Secretary of Defense, 2014), which largely examined the extent of TRICARE-covered visits to non-network providers and to emergency rooms, concluded that access to pediatric care was adequate. Likewise, the 2017 DHB report found that TRICARE largely met standards of adequacy for direct care as determined by the average days between a consult and referral appointment. However, the metrics used to evaluate pediatric access in these reports were limited. The 2017 DHB report concluded that the MHS lacked a means of comprehensively evaluating patient and family experiences systemwide and suffered from several other data-collection deficiencies. Additionally, both reports acknowledged access-related problems that occurred with PCS and other relocations, particularly for children with special or complex needs. The 2018 plan for improving pediatric care revealed that data, monitoring, and known barriers to access were the target of several MHS initiatives (DoD, 2018b). The status of these efforts had not been made publicly available as of this writing.

During this same period in which these assessments were conducted, TRICARE underwent significant changes in terms of how benefits were delivered (e.g., changes to the plans offered, reorganization under DHA) and the types of care allowed (e.g., increased opportunities to access urgent care, changes to coverage policies for autism care, increased availability of behavioral health treatment). Many of these changes were driven, in part, by a goal to improve access to care for beneficiaries; however, it was beyond the scope of this review to assess in detail how these changes have affected access to care for TRICARE-covered dependent children. Perhaps the most significant policy changes were in how DoD authorizes and pays for behavioral health care for children and adolescents. Concurrent with these policy changes were changes to how DoD monitors care access and quality. Many of these changes (if fully implemented) should facilitate more-robust analyses of access for TRICARE-covered children in the future.

Organization of This Report

Chapter Two of this report describes the objectives and methods that we employed in our own analyses. Chapters Three through Five describe the results of our analyses of the National Survey of Child Health (NSCH) and the Blue Star Families' Military Family Lifestyle Survey (MFLS). Using these data, we analyzed a variety of access experiences among TRICARE-covered families, comparing them externally with the experiences of civilian populations and internally among different groups of TRICARE beneficiaries across the TRICARE system. We present results both overall (Chapter Three) and among children with SHCN (Chapter Four), who are especially vulnerable to access barriers. Finally, we examine the role that service-related relocations might play in pediatric access experiences (Chapter Five). Chapter Six presents our conclusions and recommendations.

CHAPTER TWO

Study Objective and Overview of Methods

The goal of our study was to use readily available secondary data to evaluate the experiences of TRICARE-covered families in accessing pediatric care. We first explored how the pediatric care experiences of TRICARE-covered military families compared with those of their civilian counterparts. Second, we examined how the experiences of TRICARE-covered families varied across the MHS. Third, we assessed how the particular experiences of families of children with SHCN compared with other groups both within and outside the TRICARE system. Fourth, we examined the impact that frequent relocations have on access to pediatric care. Finally, we developed recommendations for DHA to improve monitoring and access to care for children covered by TRICARE.

Data Sources

TRICARE has not comprehensively measured pediatric patient experience data on access and quality since the 2010 HCSDB. Therefore, we used secondary data sources to conduct our analysis. Our principal data were the 2016–2018 years of the NSCH, a survey conducted by the U.S. Census Bureau on the physical and emotional health of U.S. children from birth to 17 years old (U.S. Census Bureau, undated). We supplemented our analysis with data from the 2018 MFLS, conducted by Blue Star Families, a nonprofit organization that supports military families (Blue Star Families, undated). Blue Star Families conducts this annual survey of its nearly 150,000 members and other military families via internet outreach. In the following sections, we briefly describe the features of each data set in more detail.

National Survey of Children's Health

The NSCH is a national survey sponsored by the Health Resources and Services Administration in the U.S. Department of Health and Human Services and conducted by the U.S. Census Bureau. Parents or other caregivers complete the surveys in reference to one child who lives in the household. Over the years 2016–2018, surveys were completed for 100,916 children, 3,320 of whom were identified as having TRICARE coverage: 1,581 in 2016, 695 in 2017, and 1,044 in 2018. The survey is designed to allow researchers to merge and analyze results over several years. The overall response rate on the 2018 NSCH was 43.1 percent.

Military Family Lifestyle Survey

The MFLS is a national survey sponsored by Blue Star Families and administered by the Institute for Veterans and Military Families at Syracuse University (Blue Star Families, 2018). The annual web survey is completed by an online convenience sample of military families who are recruited via email distribution lists, social media, and outreach by partner organizations. From the 10,192 total respondents in 2018, we identified 3,915 respondents who reported having both TRICARE coverage and children younger than 18. A total sample size was indeterminable, given non–probability-based methods of outreach; therefore, a response rate could not be calculated.

Where possible, we compared the sociodemographic characteristics of each of these samples with official statistics from DoD. Table 2.1 shows that the age distribution of the NSCH sample of TRICARE-covered children closely matched that of the MHS population. The sample of TRICARE-covered children in the NSCH was also similar to the total military force in terms of race and ethnicity.

Child demographics were not available in the MFLS data set, so we compared the distribution of military service branch, insurance type, and the geographic location of parent/caregiver respondents with that of the overall MHS population (Table 2.2). MFLS respondents were more likely to be in the Marine Corps and less likely to be in the

Table 2.1
Representativeness of TRICARE-Covered Children in the NSCH Sample

Characteristic	2017–2018 NSCH (%)	2018 DoD Statistics (%)[a]
Age		
0–4	28	29
5–14	53	55
15–17	18	16
Race		
White alone	67	71
Black	16	17
Asian	3	4
Other	14	8
Ethnicity		
Not Hispanic or Latino	81	85
Hispanic or Latino	19	15

SOURCES: U.S. Census Bureau, undated; DHA, 2019; DoD, 2018a; analysis of 2017–2018 NSCH data, weighted to match the demographics of the U.S. Census Bureau's 2016–2017 American Community Survey.

[a] Statistics on child age reflect the MHS population in the Defense Enrollment Eligibility Reporting System (DEERS). Statistics on race reflect all force members (not children) as reported in the 2018 Profile of the Military Community (DoD, 2018a).

Army than the broader MHS population. They were also more likely to be enrolled in TRICARE Prime. We compared the geographic distribution of 2018 MFLS respondents with that of the total MHS population in 2018. Although the MFLS sample generally showed a similar geographic composition to the MHS population, California, Virginia, and Hawaii were overrepresented, and Texas, Florida, Georgia, and South Carolina were underrepresented. (See Figure A.1 in the appendix.)

Table 2.2
Representativeness of the MFLS

Characteristic	MFLS Sample (%)	Eligible TRICARE Beneficiaries (%)
Service branch		
Army	35	41
Navy	22	21
Air Force	24	27
Marine Corps	14	8
Other	5	3
TRICARE Plan		
Prime	78	65
Select	14	33
Unenrolled/other	7	2

SOURCES: Blue Star Families, 2018; DHA, 2019.

NOTE: The TRICARE Prime category includes Prime enrollees whose care is received through primary care managers (PCMs) at MTFs and network PCMs, as well as enrollees in Prime Remote and the US Family Health Plan.

Specific Measures

Pediatric Experience Outcomes
National Survey of Children's Health

We evaluated survey responses for 16 outcomes related to accessing health care across six domains: usual source of care, specialist care, getting needed care, care coordination, insurance coverage and affordability, and patient-centeredness. For the purposes of our analysis, we grouped question responses with more than two categories into binary positive and negative responses for logistic regressions. In a few instances, question wording and response options varied slightly between the 2016–2017 and 2018 survey years. We did not observe large differences in responses between years when question wording changed, but we adjusted for the survey year in our models to mitigate the impact of wording changes or other design effects on our results. Table A.1 in the appendix shows precise question wording in each year and how they were merged, where applicable. One outcome, a measure of provider responsiveness to caregiver concerns, was a combined measure with three questions about whether a child's providers discussed treatment options, made it easy to raise concerns about recommendations, and included the caregiver in treatment decisions. One domain, "getting needed care" applied to medical, dental, and vision care; given that TRICARE does not include dental or vision benefits for family members (who may voluntarily enroll in separate TRICARE dental or Federal Employees Vision Insurance plans), this might affect comparisons with public insurance, under which dental and vision coverage are typically required.

Military Family Lifestyle Survey

We evaluated survey responses for four outcomes. Two of the outcomes related directly to experiences accessing pediatric care: timeliness in seeing a medical provider when a child needed care and the timeliness in obtaining a referral when a child required one, with four response categories ranging from strongly disagree to strongly agree. The two other outcomes related to overall satisfaction with access to care and the quality of providers, with four response categories ranging from extremely dissatisfied to extremely satisfied.

Insurance Coverage
National Survey of Children's Health

We categorized NSCH respondents based on the type of health insurance coverage that caregivers reported that their child had at the time the survey was completed (point-in-time coverage). Consistent with prior research (Seshadri et al., 2019), we classified all respondents as having TRICARE if they reported TRICARE coverage, regardless of any additional coverage they might have reported. A significant number of children reported to have TRICARE were also reported to have coverage "through a current or former employer or union," which may reflect service members or spouses employed by the military.

To investigate how insurance specification influenced our results, we conducted a sensitivity test for all our models with insurance as the main outcome, restricting our sample to only respondents who identified a single source of insurance. Point estimates were generally unaffected, although variance was higher due to the smaller sample size. (See Tables A.5 and A.6 in the appendix for these results.) We classified remaining respondents as commercially insured if they reported employer-sponsored, union, or direct-purchase insurance. Publicly insured respondents were those with Medicaid or another government assistance plan for people with low incomes or a disability, regardless of other insurance. We classified children as uninsured if caregivers reported that the child had no insurance at the time of the survey. Respondents who reported coverage through the Indian Health Service or who specified that they had a type of health insurance not included among the given options were specified as "other." These respondents were retained in our models for their contribution to variable covariance, but we exclude them from the results tables in this report due to the low substantive value of a mixed category.

Military Family Lifestyle Survey

MFLS respondents were placed into TRICARE insurance plan groups according to self-reported plan. Of 12 listed TRICARE plans, we grouped respondents into TRICARE Prime receiving care at MTFs, TRICARE Prime with a PCM (including TRICARE Remote and US Family Health Plan, which use Prime benefits and non-MTF PCMs), and TRICARE Select. Respondents with overseas plans, TRICARE for Life (Medicare wraparound coverage), and TRICARE Young Adult were excluded from comparisons of TRICARE coverage categories due to small sample sizes.

Analysis

We evaluated the relative likelihood of various pediatric access experience outcomes using multivariable logistic regressions. More detail about model specification and included adjustors can be found in the "Approach" sections of the respective chapters in which those analyses appear. All our analyses were cross-sectional, with NSCH analyses performed on the merged years 2016–2018. NSCH analyses, including regressions, were conducted using sample weights included in the public data set using statistical packages designed to account for survey data with complex sampling designs in the estimation of standard errors.

Adjusting for Multiple Comparisons

With every additional test performed, the likelihood of results being incorrectly presented as statistically significant ("false positives") increases. There are various adjustments to significance tests to account for multiple comparisons, although they can significantly increase the likelihood of results being incorrectly presented as null ("false negatives") and do not account for instances in which test results are correlated, as is likely the case for pediatric access outcomes. Additionally, guidance on what should be considered a part of a family of comparisons that need to be adjusted is ambiguous, inconsistently applied, and leads to potentially arbitrary determinations of the number of tests on which a particular adjustment is based, causing potentially misleading perceptions of the robustness of statistical findings (Feise, 2002). Given the largely exploratory nature of the estimates in this report and the high number of tests performed, we conducted tests of significance without adjusting for multiple comparisons (Althouse, 2016; Perneger, 1998; Rothman, 1990). Although we aimed to present all results with appropriate caution and context, we also note the number of false positive results we would expect, given the significance threshold and the number of tests performed, to assist in interpreting the results.

Limitations

We highlight several general limitations of the data used in this study. First, source of health insurance in the data sets was self-reported, and, therefore, relevant results are subject to misclassification error. If respondents mistakenly self-identified as having or not having TRICARE in a way that is uncorrelated with access outcomes, this would likely result in an attenuation of any true underlying differences. Second, our results are based on a national sample and an internet convenience sample that were not designed to be representative of the TRICARE population. In the case of the NSCH, as shown in Table 2.1, the demographics of TRICARE-covered children were consistent with available DoD statistics on relevant populations. Geographic differences between TRICARE and the general population in this sample were also consistent with the distribution of service members in the United States (data not shown). As discussed, data from the MFLS came from an internet convenience sample and therefore are likely not representative of the MHS population to the extent that outreach for the survey did not reach all military families. Respondents may have differentially responded to or completed the MFLS based on demographic or other characteristics. Given the high risk of a lack of representativeness in the MFLS, confirmed for some demographics in Table 2.2, we present only relative differences between comparison groups. An additional limitation is the risk of recall bias in survey responses. Retrospective reporting of past events on a survey is error-prone and subject to known biases that could systematically affect the validity of some responses.

CHAPTER THREE

Evaluation of Access to Care Among TRICARE-Covered Children

In this chapter we present two analyses: (1) our analysis of the 2016–2018 NSCH to compare the experiences of caregivers of TRICARE-covered children with those of caregivers of children in other insurance groups and (2) our analysis of the 2018 MLFS to compare the experiences of different groups of caregivers of children covered by TRICARE.

Approach

As described in Chapter One, we were unable to identify recent standardized metrics of pediatric access experiences in the available and readily accessible TRICARE data that could be applied to the entire TRICARE population under age 18. Therefore, we were limited in using MHS data to evaluate how TRICARE performed relative to other insurance or health systems in terms of pediatric access experiences. Instead, we evaluated the access experiences of caregivers of TRICARE-covered children using data from the 2016–2018 years of the NSCH and the 2018 MFLS. We assessed the overall performance of TRICARE according to caregiver experiences accessing pediatric care by comparing the experiences of caregivers of TRICARE-covered children with those of caregivers of children with other types of insurance and without any insurance. Within TRICARE, we compared experiences with pediatric health care access among active-duty service members and non–active-duty service members, across TRICARE insurance plan groupings (TRICARE Prime with MTF PCM, TRICARE Prime with private PCM, and TRICARE Select), and across service branches (Army, Navy, Air Force, and Marine Corps).

Active-Duty Status
National Survey of Children's Health

Since 2017, the annual NSCH has asked caregivers whether they or another primary caregiver has ever served on active duty in the U.S. armed forces, reserves, or National Guard. Respondents can indicate whether they are on active duty at the time of the survey, were on active duty only for training in the reserves or National Guard, or were on active duty in the past but not at the time of the survey. If the respondent or another caregiver was identified as being on active duty at the time of the survey, we categorized the respondent as active duty.[1]

Military Family Lifestyle Survey

The MFLS asks respondents whether a service member or spouse/domestic partner is currently on active duty, was on active duty in the past, was never on active duty except for initial or basic training, or had never served on active duty. Unlike the NSCH question on active-duty status, the MFLS clarifies that active duty includes activated reserve and National Guard personnel.

Analysis
National Survey of Children's Health

We used multivariable logistic regression models to estimate the likelihood of each pediatric access outcome by insurance type. Independent variables included insurance type, sex, age, income, race, census region, whether the child had SHCN, whether the child ever had a mental health diagnosis, and survey year. We selected these variables based on their inclusion in prior studies on this topic (Seshadri et al., 2019). We report results from these models as average adjusted predicted probabilities by insurance category. To compare the active-duty and

---

[1] Service members in the reserve component (including National Guard) may not define *active duty* the same way as official DoD policy. This phrase is sometimes understood to mean full-time military service members (not reserve or national guard). Therefore, some activated members of the reserve component may have been misclassified in our measure.

non–active-duty categories, we used logistic regressions adjusting only for survey year. All regressions were performed using multiply imputed data sets from the U.S. Census Bureau to account for missing income data. To prevent loss of information in the estimation of these models, we retained the "other" insurance category; however, given the heterogeneity of the category estimates on this variable, those results are likely not substantively meaningful and are not presented in our results. Additionally, there is a possibility that many who report "other" insurance represented misclassifications of other insurance categories considered in our analysis. Therefore, as a robustness check, we reran all analyses of insurance type after excluding the "other" category from the data, and there were no meaningful changes to our results.

Military Family Lifestyle Survey

We used multivariable logistic regression models to estimate the likelihood of each pediatric access outcome by TRICARE plan grouping (TRICARE Prime with a PCM at an MTF, TRICARE Prime with a network PCM, and TRICARE Select) and by military service branch. Independent variables included military service branch, TRICARE plan, sex, race/ethnicity, education, income, census region, self-reported SHCN status, and mental health counseling in the past year (any family member). Given that the MFLS uses a convenience sample that is unlikely to be representative of the general military population, we do not report predicted probabilities from these data. Instead, we calculated average marginal effects of the comparison groups relative to a reference category (the Army) or the average difference, over the sample, in the likelihood of each outcome in each comparison group when compared with a reference category. Given the inconsistency between the MFLS and the NSCH in how *active duty* was defined and the fact that the large majority of MFLS respondents indicated that they were currently active, we did not conduct that analysis for the MFLS data.

Results

Our insurance groupings showed substantial differences in socio-demographic characteristics (Table 3.1). Compared with the care-

Table 3.1
Respondent Characteristics, by Insurance Type

Characteristic	Insurance Type (%)				
	All	TRICARE	Commercial	Public	None
Number in sample	100,916	3,320	68,663	21,955	3,632
Weighted sample proportion	100	2	54	34	6
Demographic characteristics					
Sex					
Male	51	53	51	52	52
Female	49	47	49	48	48
Age (years)					
0–5	32	33	32	34	26
6–12	39	37	39	41	40
13–17	28	30	29	25	34
Race/ethnicity					
Non-Hispanic white	51	55	65	34	34
Non-Hispanic black	13	15	8	21	15
Hispanic	25	19	16	36	41
Other	11	11	11	9	10
Family income level (% of federal poverty level)					
Low (< 133%)	29	15	8	59	47
Middle (133–400%)	40	51	42	36	42
High (> 400%)	30	34	50	5	11
Census region					
Midwest	16	7	18	15	11
Northeast	21	13	24	19	17
South	39	54	34	42	52
West	24	25	24	24	20

Table 3.1—Continued

Characteristic	Insurance Type (%)				
	All	TRICARE	Commercial	Public	None
Education					
Less than high school	9	2	2	17	27
High school	19	8	10	34	29
More than high school	71	91	88	49	44
Risk factors					
SHCN					
Yes	19	21	16	25	12
No	81	79	84	75	88
Ever had MBHCN					
Yes	81	79	83	77	84
No	19	21	16	23	16
Rate of address changes since child's birth					
Never moved	34	18	40	27	33
At least 1 move, less than 1 every 2 years	56	61	54	58	57
More than 1 move every 2 years	10	21	6	15	11

SOURCE: Analysis of 2016–2018 NSCH data.

NOTES: Sample numbers reflect unweighted numbers of responses, while percentages are weighted to reflect sampling design and demographics from the U.S. Census Bureau's 2015–2017 American Community Survey. Differences among insurance groups using chi-squared tests were statistically significant in all sociodemographic groups except sex. Roughly 4 percent of respondents indicated that their child was covered by some other type of insurance and are excluded from the table.

givers of all other children nationally, a lower proportion of caregivers of TRICARE-covered children were low-income (15 percent had incomes less than 133 percent of the federal poverty level versus 29 percent nationally), and a higher proportion had greater than a high school degree (91 percent versus 71 percent nationally) and lived in the southern region of the United States (54 percent versus 39 percent nationally). Additionally, TRICARE-covered children changed home addresses considerably more frequently than children nationally (21 percent changed address more than once every two years, compared with 10 percent nationally). A higher proportion of caregivers of publicly insured and uninsured children were nonwhite, low-income, and had low education. Caregivers of commercially insured children were less racially diverse, had higher incomes, and changed addresses at a lower rate than caregivers of children nationally.

Access to Care under TRICARE Compared with Other Coverage Groups

Table 3.2 shows model-adjusted average predicted probabilities of pediatric access experiences among caregivers of TRICARE-covered children compared with their counterparts in other coverage groups.

Usual Source of Care

Caregivers of TRICARE-covered children and those of children with commercial and public insurance plans were similarly likely to report having a usual place of care for their children in case of illness (82 percent versus 83 percent for commercial insurance and 79 percent for public insurance) and for routine preventive care (95 percent versus 95 percent for commercial insurance and 92 percent for public insurance). Fewer caregivers of TRICARE-covered children reported having at least one person they considered their child's personal doctor or nurse than did those with commercial insurance or public insurance (68 percent versus 76 percent for commercial insurance and 72 percent for public insurance).

Referral to Specialist Care

Caregivers of TRICARE-covered children were significantly more likely than those in other insurance categories to report needing a

Table 3.2
Pediatric Access Experiences, by Insurance Type

Access Category	TRICARE (reference)	Commercial	Public	None
	Insurance Type (%)			
Number in sample	3,320	68,663	21,955	3,632
Usual source of care				
Has usual source of care when child is sick	82	83	79*	63***
Has usual source of care for child's routine preventive care	95	95	92**	75***
Caregiver thinks of one or more persons as child's doctor or nurse	68	76***	72*	53***
Specialist care (in past year)				
Child needed referral	26	17***	20***	14***
Had difficulty getting a referral	26	15***	23	36
Had difficulty getting mental health treatment	44	48	42	52
Had difficulty getting specialist care	28	22	28	34
Getting needed care (in past year)				
Child needed care but did not receive it	3	2	3	10***
Care coordination (in past year)				
Received help coordinating care	26	18***	19***	15***
Could have used more help coordinating care	9	6*	9	7
Insurance coverage and affordability				
Health insurance usually covers child's health care needs	95	92*	95	—
Health insurance usually allows child to see health care provider	96	96	97	—
Health insurance usually covers child's MBHCN	80	65***	77	—

Table 3.2—Continued

Access Category	Insurance Type (%)			
	TRICARE (reference)	Commercial	Public	None
Had problems paying health care bills in past year	10	15**	15**	23***
Patient-centeredness (in past year)				
Usually frustrated getting health care services	19	13***	19	28***
Health care providers usually responsive to concerns	90	89	83*	81*

SOURCE: Analysis of 2016–2018 NSCH data.

NOTES: All percentages represent the average predicted probabilities, adjusted for sociodemographics. Tests of significance performed using Wald tests of coefficients relative to the reference category. In 61 tests, we would expect three significant results due to chance alone at $p < 0.05$, 0.6 significant results at $p < 0.01$, and 0.06 significant results at $p < 0.001$, assuming all tests are independent. * $p < 0.05$, ** $p < 0.01$, *** $p < 0.001$.

referral to see a doctor in the past year. This likely stems from the high proportion of TRICARE-covered families enrolled in its HMO option (TRICARE Prime) compared with HMO enrollment among those with commercial insurance (Kongstvedt, 2013). A quarter (26 percent) of caregivers of TRICARE-covered children needed a referral, compared with 17 percent in commercial plans and 20 percent in public plans. Among children who needed a referral, caregivers of TRICARE-covered children reported more difficulty obtaining the referral than those of commercially covered children (26 percent versus 15 percent).

Specialty care—especially mental health care—was difficult to obtain for many TRICARE families, although we did not find evidence that it was any more difficult for TRICARE-covered children to receive needed mental health or specialist care than children in any other insurance category. Among children who had seen a specialist or needed to see a specialist (excluding mental health) in the year prior to the survey, 28 percent of caregivers of TRICARE-covered children reported at least some difficulty getting care. Among caregivers of TRICARE-covered children who either received treatment or needed to receive treatment from a mental health professional in the previous year, 44 percent reported at least some difficulty getting needed mental health treatment or counseling.

Getting Needed Care

Caregivers of TRICARE-covered children and their counterparts in other coverage categories reported similar rates of not getting needed health care. Among TRICARE-covered children, 3 percent reportedly did not receive needed health care in the prior year, compared with 2 percent with commercial insurance, 3 percent with public insurance, and 10 percent of uninsured children.

Care Coordination

Survey responses on care coordination indicated that TRICARE-covered children may have more access to care coordination services than children with other insurance types, but this assistance may not compensate for differences in the need for these services. Caregivers of TRICARE-covered children were more likely than caregivers in the commercially and publicly insured categories to report having someone to help with care coordination (26 percent versus 18 percent and 19 percent, respectively). However, caregivers of TRICARE-covered children were more likely than commercially insured caregivers to report feeling like they needed more help coordinating their child's care (9 percent versus 6 percent).

Insurance Coverage and Affordability

The large majority of caregivers in every insurance category felt that their insurance offered adequate coverage overall. Ninety-five percent of caregivers of TRICARE-covered children reported that their insurance benefits and coverage "usually" or "always" met their child's needs, which was higher than for commercially insured children (92 percent) and equal to publicly insured children (95 percent). Among children who received mental or behavioral health services, 80 percent of TRICARE caregivers reported that their insurance usually or always met their child's mental or behavioral health needs, which, again, was higher than in the commercially insured category (65 percent) and similar to publicly insured children (77 percent). Caregivers across all insurance types generally felt that their insurance allowed their children to see needed health care providers.

Families of TRICARE-covered children were less likely to report problems paying for their child's health care bills than those in other coverage categories. Around 10 percent of caregivers of TRICARE-covered children reported problems paying for medical bills; rates were 15 percent of commercially insured, 15 percent of publicly insured, and 23 percent of uninsured children.

Patient-Centeredness

Caregivers of TRICARE-covered children reported that health care providers were usually responsive to their concerns and included them in decisionmaking. Ninety percent of caregivers of TRICARE-covered children and 89 percent of caregivers of commercially insured children reported that their child's health care providers in the prior year were usually or always responsive, compared with 83 percent of those whose children were publicly insured and 81 percent of those whose children were uninsured.

Caregivers of TRICARE-covered children reported higher degrees of frustration getting services than those of commercially insured children and similar degrees of frustration as those of publicly insured children. Nineteen percent of TRICARE caregivers reported being usually or always frustrated getting services, compared with 13 percent of caregivers of commercially insured children and 19 percent of caregivers of publicly insured children. Caregivers of uninsured children reported the highest degree of frustration, at 28 percent.

Evaluating Access to Care under TRICARE
Access by Active-Duty Status

Among TRICARE beneficiaries, the health insurance circumstances and options of families of active-duty service members differed from those of families with non–active-duty service members in ways that may have affected access experiences. Because some insurance options are available only to active-duty service members, the health insurance options for reserve-component members may be in fluctuation as they cycle in and out of activation. We used the NSCH to compare TRICARE families with caregivers on active duty with families without a caregiver on active duty. Generally, families with an active-duty caregiver reported better pediatric access experiences than those not on active duty (Table 3.3).

For routine care, active-duty families were more likely to report a usual source of care when sick (88 percent versus 80 percent) Active-duty families also reported less difficulty obtaining specialist care

Table 3.3
Pediatric Access Experiences, by Active-Duty Status

Access Category	Active-Duty Status at Time of Survey (%)	
	Not Active Duty	Active Duty
Number in sample	1,010	698
Usual source of care		
Has usual source of care when child is sick	80	88*
Has usual source of care for child's routine preventive care	95	97
Caregiver thinks of one or more persons as child's doctor or nurse	71	66
Specialist care (in past year)		
Child needed referral	28	28
Had difficulty getting a referral	23	34
Had difficulty getting mental health treatment	53	40
Had difficulty getting specialist care	34	17*
Getting needed care (in past year)		
Child needed care but did not receive it	5	1**
Care coordination (in past year)		
Received help coordinating care	24	34
Could have used more help coordinating care	10	8

Table 3.3—Continued

Access Category	Active-Duty Status at Time of Survey (%)	
	Not Active Duty	Active Duty
Insurance coverage and affordability		
Health insurance usually covers child's health care needs	92	98*
Health insurance usually allows child to see health care provider	95	97
Health insurance usually covers child's MBHCN	75	91*
Had problems paying health care bills in past year	14	6*
Patient-centeredness (in past year)		
Usually frustrated getting health care services	22	17
Health care providers usually responsive to concerns	91	85

SOURCE: Analysis of 2017–2018 NSCH data. The 2016 data set was excluded because it did not include active-duty status.

NOTES: The table shows the average predicted probability of each outcome by active-duty status, adjusted for survey year. Tests of significance performed using Wald tests of coefficients relative to the reference category. In 16 tests, we would expect less than one significant result due to chance alone at $p < 0.05$ and less than 0.2 significant results at $p < 0.01$, assuming all tests are independent. * $p < 0.05$, ** $p < 0.01$.

(17 percent versus 34 percent) and were substantially more likely to report adequate coverage for MBHCN than non–active-duty families (91 percent versus 75 percent). Finally, active-duty families were less likely to report not getting needed care (1 percent versus 5 percent) and were less likely to report having trouble paying health care bills (6 percent versus 14 percent).

Access by TRICARE Plan

TRICARE beneficiaries can be enrolled in one of several types of TRI-CARE plans, depending on eligibility. Generally, dependents of service members can be enrolled in either an HMO-type plan known as

TRICARE Prime or a PPO-type plan known as TRICARE Select. Family members in TRICARE Prime have lower cost-sharing than those in TRICARE Select but typically must be seen for specialty care at an MTF and require prior authorization and a referral from a PCM for most nonroutine care. Family members in TRICARE Select have higher cost-sharing but more flexibility in providers and do not need referrals to see specialists. TRICARE Prime family members can choose a PCM at an MTF or a network (civilian) PCM in the community. In FY 2018, 66 percent of eligible children under age 18 were covered by TRICARE Prime, and 32 percent were covered by TRICARE Select (DHA, 2019).

Data on TRICARE plans were not available in the NSCH, but the MFLS asked respondents to report their TRICARE plan (see Table A.2 in the appendix). Caregivers with TRICARE Prime and a PCM at an MTF reported more issues seeing a pediatric medical provider in a reasonable amount of time than those in TRICARE Prime with a network PCM or in TRICARE Select (Table 3.4). Compared with TRICARE Prime with a PCM at an MTF, TRICARE Prime enrollees with a network PCM were, on average, 7.3 percentage points more likely to agree that they received timely pediatric care when it was needed, compared with 10.0 percentage points for TRICARE Select. Caregivers with TRICARE Prime with a network PCM and TRICARE Select were also 12.2 and 20.9 percentage points more likely, respectively, than those with TRICARE Prime and a PCM at an MTF to report satisfaction with the overall ease of access and timeliness of their health care (for all covered family members).

Access by Service Branch

Over the study period, MTFs were mostly managed and operated by the military services. We compared pediatric access experiences across branches of service, using data from the MFLS. (See Table A.3 in the appendix for detailed observations by service branch.) Pediatric access experiences and overall satisfaction were generally consistent across the Army, Navy, and Marine Corps (Table 3.5). Air Force respondents tended to report somewhat worse pediatric access and overall satisfaction with care than Army and Navy respondents. For example, on aver-

Table 3.4
Average Marginal Effects of TRICARE Insurance Type Compared with TRICARE Prime and a PCM at an MTF

Access Category	TRICARE Plan/Care Setting (%)		
	TRICARE Prime (PCM at MTF)	TRICARE Prime (Network PCM)	TRICARE Select
Number in sample	2,067	1,003	553
Pediatric access experiences			
Received timely pediatric care when needed (73% agree overall)	(Reference)	+7.3***	+10.0***
Received timely pediatric referrals when needed (69% agree overall)	(Reference)	+1.8	–1.4
Overall satisfaction			
Ease and timeliness of access (72% satisfied overall)	(Reference)	+12.2***	+20.9***
Quality of providers (78% satisfied overall)	(Reference)	+5.8***	+10.9***

SOURCE: Analysis of MFLS data.

NOTES: The table shows average marginal effects, adjusted for sociodemographics, of different insurance categories relative to the reference (TRICARE Prime with a PCM at an MTF). Numbers express, on average, how much more or less likely an individual in the sample would be to give the response if recategorized from the reference category to the new category. For example, on average, we expect caregivers of children enrolled in TRICARE Select to be 10 percentage points more likely to agree that the child received timely pediatric care when needed compared with TRICARE Prime (PCM at MTF). Satisfaction outcomes apply to care for all members of families with children under age 18, not just pediatric care. In eight tests, we would expect less than 0.01 significant results due to chance alone at $p < 0.001$, assuming all tests are independent. *** $p < 0.001$.

age, Air Force respondents were 6.6 percentage points less likely to agree that they received timely pediatric care when needed, 4.6 percentage points less likely to agree that they received timely pediatric referrals when needed, 6.2 percentage points less likely to be satisfied with the ease and timeliness of access to care, and 4.1 percentage points less likely to be satisfied with the quality of providers.

Access by Region

We also compared access experiences among TRICARE families across U.S. geographic census divisions, with Alaska and Hawaii included as separate categories. The Pacific and Mountain divisions tended to perform worse than other regions across several outcomes, including receiving timely pediatric care when needed and receiving timely pediatric referrals when needed (data not shown).

Table 3.5
Average Marginal Effects of Military Service Branch Compared with the Army

| Access Category | Military Service Branch (%) | | | |
	Army	Navy	Air Force	Marine Corps
Number in sample	1,383	866	948	533
Pediatric access experiences				
Received timely pediatric care when needed (73% agree overall)	(Reference)	+0.1	−6.6***	−1.3
Received timely pediatric referrals when needed (69% agree overall)	(Reference)	+2.3	−4.6*	−2.7
Overall satisfaction				
Ease and timeliness of access (72% satisfied overall)	(Reference)	+0.1	−6.2**	−4.5
Quality of providers (78% satisfied overall)	(Reference)	+1.2	−4.1*	−3.5

SOURCE: Analysis of MFLS data.

NOTES: Table shows average marginal effects, adjusted for sociodemographics, of military service branch categories relative to the reference (the Army). Numbers express, on average, how much more or less likely an individual in the sample would be to give the response if recategorized from the reference category to the new category. Satisfaction outcomes apply to care for all members of families with children under age 18, not just pediatric care. In 12 tests, we would expect less than one significant result due to chance alone at $p < 0.05$, less than 0.2 significant results at $p < 0.01$, and less than 0.02 significant results at $p < 0.001$, assuming all tests are independent. * $p < 0.05$, ** $p < 0.01$, *** $p < 0.001$.

Summary

Using data from the 2016–2018 years of the NSCH and the 2018 MFLS, we evaluated the access experiences of TRICARE-covered children relative to children covered by other insurance types and with no insurance. Caregivers of TRICARE-covered children were less likely to have one person they considered their child's personal doctor or nurse, were more likely to need referrals, and reported greater difficulty getting a referral when needed than those with commercial or public insurance. Although the majority of caregivers found that their insurance coverage was adequate, caregivers of TRICARE-covered children were more likely to report having coverage for MBHCN and less likely to report problems paying for care than those of children with commercial and public insurance. Caregivers of children with TRICARE also reported similar responsiveness of care as those with commercial insurance and moderately higher responsiveness than those with public insurance.

Additionally, we performed within-TRICARE comparisons by active-duty status across TRICARE plan groupings and service branches. We found that active-duty families were more likely to report a usual source of care when sick, had less difficulty obtaining specialty care, and were more likely to report adequate coverage for MBHCN than non–active-duty families. Active-duty families were less likely to report not getting needed care and having trouble paying health care bills. Looking specifically at TRICARE insurance types, respondents with TRICARE Prime with a network PCM and those with TRICARE Select were more likely than those with TRICARE Prime with a PCM at an MTF to agree that they received timely pediatric care when it was needed. Caregivers with TRICARE Prime with a network PCM and those with TRICARE Select were also more likely than those with a TRICARE PCM at an MTF to report satisfaction with the overall ease of access and timeliness of their health care.

We found that pediatric access experiences and overall satisfaction were generally consistent across the Army, Navy, and Marine Corps but worse for Air Force respondents. Air Force respondents were less likely to agree that they received timely pediatric care when needed, less likely to agree that they received timely pediatric referrals when needed, less likely to be satisfied with the ease and timeliness of access to care, and less likely to be satisfied with the quality of providers.

CHAPTER FOUR

Children with Special Health Care Needs

The importance of having access to quality health care increases as medical, mental, and behavioral health needs increase (Berry et al., 2015). A 2004 study found that 23 percent of children covered by TRICARE had SHCN. These children had five times as many admissions and spent ten times as many days in the hospital as children without SHCN, and they accounted for half of outpatient visits (Williams et al., 2004). The burdens of poor access multiply with higher utilization, and the health consequences of any care delayed or forgone are more severe. As a result, the access and quality experiences of families with children with SHCN can suffer. Despite these risks, children with SHCN are often not given the support they need (Newacheck et al., 2000). A 2018 national study of children with SHCN found that their caregivers reported worse access to medical homes, which can provide needed consistency, coordination, and community services (Lichstein, Ghandour, and Mann, 2018). A 2019 analysis of MEPS data suggested that access experiences of TRICARE-covered children with high medical complexity were worse than among children without SHCN, identifying gaps in access experiences among TRICARE-covered children with behavioral health diagnoses (Seshadri et al., 2019). However, DHA questioned these findings (Adirim, Hisle-Gorman, and Klein, 2019). To further examine this potential area of need, we extended our analysis to TRICARE-covered children with SHCN.

Approach

Defining Special Health Care Needs

There is no standard way of defining SHCN. One means of identifying children with SHCN in the MHS is through their enrollment in programs that provide assistance to designated groups. One such program is the EFMP, which uses provider-centric eligibility criteria, with a nurse reviewing a patient's files, and is administered by each of the military services through offices located at MTFs. Service members can enroll in the EFMP if a family member requires special medical services for a chronic condition, is being seen by a specialist on an ongoing basis, has significant behavioral health concerns, or receives early intervention or special education services. However, because not all military families with SHCN enroll in the EFMP, there is no database or registry in the MHS that can identify all TRICARE families with SHCN (Military OneSource, 2020; National Institutes of Health, 2014). In FY 2016, 104,677 family members across the services were enrolled in the EFMP, accounting for roughly 5 percent of TRICARE-eligible children (U.S. Government Accountability Office [GAO], 2018). More recently, the MHS has used the pediatric medical complexity algorithm (DHA, 2017)—an emerging indicator of pediatric medical complexity that uses International Classification of Diseases (ICD) codes—as a basis for comparing and benchmarking TRICARE to the civilian population.[1] Using this algorithm, DHA reported that, in 2015, 17 percent of children MHS-wide had a non-complex chronic condition, while 6 percent had a complex chronic condition (DHA, 2017).

To identify TRICARE families with SHCN in the NSCH data, we used a standardized five-item screening tool developed by the Child and Adolescent Health Measurement Initiative based on a definition of SHCN developed by the Maternal and Child Health Bureau of the Health Resources and Services Administration. This screening tool has consistently been validated to identify subsets of

---

[1]   At the time of its adoption, the algorithm used the ninth edition of the ICD (ICD-9); it now uses the tenth (ICD-10).

children with chronic conditions that need or use more care and have heightened needs for various forms of assistance (Bethell et al., 2015). The screening questions asked whether the child (1) was limited in their ability to perform age-appropriate activities; (2) needed or used prescription medications (aside from vitamins); (3) needed or used specialized therapies; (4) had an uncommon need for medical, mental health, or educational services; or (5) needed or received treatment or counseling for emotional, developmental, or behavioral problems. A child was identified as having SHCN if their caregiver responded affirmatively to one of the five health consequences and reported that the consequence was due to an underlying medical, behavioral, or other health condition that had lasted or was expected to last more than 12 months. Roughly 20 percent of TRICARE-covered children in our sample were identified as having SHCN through this screener, which corresponded to roughly 17 percent of MHS-enrolled children in 2015 with a noncomplex chronic condition.

We also identified families with children with MBHCN using a series of NSCH questions asking whether a caregiver had ever been told by a health care provider that their child had one of a list of behavioral or developmental health conditions. (See the appendix for a list of conditions.) Due to sample limitations, we used a broad definition of MBHCN. We categorized caregivers as having a child with MBHCN if they answered affirmatively to at least one of these questions or indicated that they had been told by a health care provider that their child had "any other mental health condition." Roughly 21 percent of TRICARE-covered children in our sample were identified as having such a need.

The MFLS identifies respondents with special needs using a single self-reported question: "Do you have a child(ren) with special needs?" Roughly 20 percent of MFLS respondents answered "yes" to this question.

Analysis

To compare the access experiences of TRICARE-covered children with SHCN or MBHCN and those without these needs, we used multivariable logistic regressions on NSCH data to estimate the likelihood of each pediatric access outcome, adjusting only for survey year. We did not include analyses with full sociodemographic controls because the estimates lacked precision due to sample size. Unadjusted results for this comparison are nonetheless valuable to understanding how access to pediatric care differs between these populations; however, these differences may not be caused by SHCN status. In robustness checks with full sociodemographic controls, point estimates were similar across outcomes. Analysis of MBHCN was limited to respondents with children ages 6 and older to maintain consistency with prior research on this population (Seshadri, 2019). Analysis of the joint conditions of SHCN and MBHCN among TRICARE-covered children and their association with pediatric access experiences can be found in Table A.4 in the appendix. We also analyzed access experiences as reported in the MFLS using multivariable logistic regression, adjusting for military service branch, TRICARE insurance plan, sex, race/ethnicity, education, income, census region, self-reported SHCN status, and prior mental health counseling in the past year (any family member).

To compare the experiences of children with SHCN covered by TRICARE and children with SHCN with other insurance types, we limited the NSCH sample to those with SHCN and used separate multivariable logistic regressions with the independent variables of insurance category, sex, age, income, race/ethnicity, census region, survey year, and MBHCN.

Results

Access Experiences of TRICARE-Covered Children with and Without SHCN

Table 4.1 shows that caregivers of TRICARE-covered children with SHCN reported significantly worse access experiences across several measures compared with caregivers of TRICARE-covered children without SHCN. TRICARE-covered children with SHCN had more difficulty getting referrals (37 percent versus 21 percent) and were less likely to get needed care (8 percent versus 2 percent reported

Table 4.1

Pediatric Access Experiences Among TRICARE-Covered Children with and Without Special Health Care Needs

Access Category	SHCN Status (%)	
	No SHCN	SHCN
Number in sample	2,516	804
Usual source of care		
Has usual source of care when child is sick	82	88*
Has usual source of care for child's routine preventive care	95	97
Caregiver thinks of one or more persons as child's doctor or nurse	69	72
Specialist care (in past year)		
Child needed referral	19	55***
Had difficulty getting a referral	21	37*
Had difficulty getting mental health treatment	43	46
Had difficulty getting specialist care	23	32
Getting needed care (in past year)		
Child needed care but did not receive it	2	8**
Care coordination (in past year)		
Received help coordinating care	24	33*
Could have used more help coordinating care	4	25***
Insurance coverage and affordability		
Health insurance usually covers child's health needs	96	93
Health insurance usually allows child to see health care provider	98	92**
Health insurance usually covers child's MBHCN	72	86*
Had problems paying health care bills in past year	11	16

Table 4.1—Continued

	SHCN Status (%)	
Access Category	No SHCN	SHCN
Patient-centeredness (in past year)		
Usually frustrated getting health care services	14	38***
Health care providers usually responsive to concerns	89	91

SOURCE: Analysis of 2016–2018 NSCH data.

NOTES: All percentages represent the average predicted probabilities, adjusted for sociodemographics. Tests of significance performed using Wald tests of coefficients relative to the reference category. In 16 tests, we would expect less than 1 significant results due to chance alone at $p < 0.05$, < 0.1 significant results at $p < 0.01$, and less than 0.01 significant results at $p < 0.001$, assuming all tests are independent. * $p < 0.05$, ** $p < 0.01$, *** $p < 0.001$.

not getting needed care). Caregivers of TRICARE-covered children with SHCN also reported more frustration getting care (38 percent versus 14 percent), and a higher desire for more help coordinating care (25 percent versus 4 percent).

Table 4.2 shows that MFLS respondents who reported having at least one child with SHCN were 13.5 percentage points less likely to report receiving timely care and 8.4 percentage points less likely to report receiving timely pediatric referrals than respondents without children with SHCN. Respondents with children with SHCN were also less satisfied with ease of access and the quality of their providers overall.

Access Experiences of TRICARE-Covered Children with and Without MBHCN

Accessing care for pediatric mental and behavioral health conditions can be especially challenging for families (So, McCord, and Kaminski, 2019). We therefore compared access experiences among caregivers of TRICARE-covered children with and without MBHCN. Caregivers of TRICARE-covered children who had ever had MBHCN reported no difference in accessing routine care compared with those whose

Table 4.2
Average Marginal Effects of Special Health Care Needs Versus No Special
Health Care Needs

| | SHCN Status (%) | |
Access Category	No Children with SHCN	At Least 1 Child with SHCN
Number in sample	2,688	682
Pediatric access experiences		
Received timely pediatric care when needed (73% agree overall)	(Reference)	−13.5***
Received timely pediatric referrals when needed (69% agree overall)	(Reference)	−8.4***
Overall satisfaction[a]		
Ease and timeliness of access (72% satisfied overall)	(Reference)	−5.7**
Quality of providers (78% satisfied overall)	(Reference)	−5.6**

SOURCE: Analysis of MFLS data.

NOTES: Table shows average marginal effects, adjusted for sociodemographics, of different SHCN statuses relative to the reference (no children with SHCN). Numbers express, on average, how much more or less likely an individual in the sample would be to give the response if recategorized from the reference category to the new category. For example, on average, we expect respondents with at least one child with SHCN to be 13.5 percentage points less likely to agree that their child received timely pediatric care when needed compared with respondents without children with SHCN. In four tests, we would expect less than 0.1 significant results due to chance alone at $p < 0.01$ and less than 0.01 significant results due to chance alone at $p < 0.001$, assuming all tests are independent. ** $p < 0.01$, *** $p < 0.001$.

[a] Satisfaction outcomes apply to care for all members of families with children under age 18, not just pediatric care.

children never had a MBHCN (Table 4.3). However, caregivers of TRICARE-covered children who had ever had MBHCN reported substantially more difficulty accessing specialty care, including difficulty getting referrals (38 percent versus 22 percent) and difficulty getting specialist care (39 percent versus 21 percent). Caregivers of TRICARE-covered children with MBHCN were also more likely to report not receiving care for their child when needed (7 percent versus 2 percent), frustration getting care (37 percent versus 14 percent), needing more

Table 4.3
Pediatric Access Experiences Among TRICARE-Covered Children with and Without Mental or Behavioral Health Care Needs

Access Category	MBHCN Status (%)	
	No MBHCN	MBHCN
Number in sample	2,583	736
Usual source of care		
Has usual source of care when child is sick	83	84
Has usual source of care for child's routine preventive care	96	96
Caregiver thinks of one or more persons as child's doctor or nurse	69	71
Specialist care (in past year)		
Child needed referral	21	46***
Had difficulty getting a referral	22	38*
Had difficulty getting mental health treatment	—	—
Had difficulty getting specialist care	21	39**
Getting needed care (in past year)		
Child needed care but did not receive it	2	7*
Care coordination (in past year)		
Received help coordinating care	26	27
Could have used more help coordinating care	6	21***
Insurance coverage and affordability		
Health insurance usually covers child's health needs	96	92
Health insurance usually allows child to see health care provider	98	91**
Health insurance usually covers child's MBHCN	71	87*
Had problems paying health care bills in past year	10	17*

Table 4.3—Continued

Access Category	MBHCN Status (%)	
	No MBHCN	MBHCN
Patient-centeredness (in past year)		
Usually frustrated getting health care services	14	37***
Health care providers usually responsive to concerns	90	90

SOURCE: Analysis of 2016–2018 NSCH data.

NOTES: All percentages represent the average predicted probabilities, adjusted for sociodemographics. For consistency with reporting in other studies (e.g., Seshadri, 2019), we report results by MBHCN only for children ages 6 and older. Tests of significance performed using Wald tests of coefficients relative to the reference category. In 15 tests, we would expect less than 1 significant result due to chance alone at $p < 0.05$, less than 0.1 significant results at $p < 0.01$, and less than 0.01 significant results at $p < 0.001$, assuming all tests are independent. * $p < 0.05$, ** $p < 0.01$, *** $p < 0.001$.

assistance coordinating care (21 percent versus 6 percent), and having problems paying for care (17 percent versus 10 percent). However, caregivers of TRICARE-covered children who had ever had MBHCN largely reported that their insurance covered their children's mental or behavioral health needs (87 percent).

TRICARE-covered families with *both* SHCN and MBHCN reported substantially worse access experiences than TRICARE-covered families who reported neither, including difficulty getting a referral, difficulty getting specialist care, not getting needed care, and frustration getting services (see Table A.4 in the appendix). They were also significantly more likely to report that they could have used more help coordinating care and less likely to say that their plan usually allowed them to see the doctor they wanted.

Access Experiences of Children with SHCN Covered by TRICARE Versus Other Insurance

We also compared TRICARE-covered children with SHCN and children with SHCN in other insurance groups (Table 4.4). Overall, our results revealed comparable access experiences among chil-

Table 4.4
Pediatric Access Experiences, by Insurance Type, Children with Special Health Care Needs

Access Category	Insurance Type (%)			
	TRICARE (reference)	Commercial	Public	None
Number in sample	804	13,586	7,090	680
Usual source of care				
Has usual source of care when child is sick	87	86	85	73***
Has usual source of care for child's routine preventive care	97	96	95	86***
Caregiver thinks of one or more persons as child's doctor or nurse	71	82**	80**	67
Specialist care (in past year)				
Child needed referral	54	31***	42**	38**
Had difficulty getting a referral	32	18**	27	45
Had difficulty getting mental health treatment	44	50	45	53
Had difficulty getting specialist care	31	25	31	39
Getting needed care (in past year)				
Child needed care but did not receive it	6	4	6	17**
Care Coordination (in past year)				
Received help coordinating care	32	22**	27	30
Could have used more help coordinating care	22	13***	17	14
Insurance coverage and affordability				
Health insurance usually covers child's health needs	94	88	94	—
Health insurance usually allows child to see health care provider	93	94	96	—
Health insurance usually covers child's MBHCN	84	63***	84	—

Table 4.4—Continued

Access Category	Insurance Type (%)			
	TRICARE (reference)	Commercial	Public	None
Had problems paying health care bills in last year	12	23***	21***	44***
Patient-centeredness (in past year)				
Usually frustrated getting health care services	33	26*	35	42
Health care providers usually responsive to concerns	92	88	82**	78*

SOURCE: Analysis of 2016–2018 NSCH data.

NOTES: All percentages represent average predicted probabilities, adjusted for sociodemographics. Tests of significance performed using Wald tests of coefficients relative to the reference category. In 61 tests, we would expect three significant results due to chance alone at $p < 0.05$, 0.6 significant results at $p < 0.01$, and 0.06 significant results at $p < 0.001$, assuming all tests are independent. * $p < 0.05$, ** $p < 0.01$, *** $p < 0.001$.

dren with SHCN in TRICARE relative to other insurance groups; this contrasts with prior research that has shown worse health care access and quality for TRICARE-covered children with SHCN compared with nonmilitary children (Seshadri et al., 2019). It is possible that this finding reflects relative improvements in pediatric access in TRICARE since the 2008–2015 period. Over the past decade, several policy changes may have served to expand coverage and ease access for TRICARE-covered children with SHCN, including fewer limits on mental health services and providers, reductions in cost-sharing for some preventive services, and expanded access to urgent care facilities (DHA, 2019). However, differences in question wording and methodology between the NSCH and data used in prior research mean that caution is warranted in speculating about changes in the data over time. As more data become available from MEPS and the NSCH, longitudinal analyses should be conducted to assess whether policy changes have been accompanied by systemwide improvements in pediatric experiences.

Obtaining referrals for specialists was a significant reported challenge for some caregivers of TRICARE-covered children with SHCN during the study period. The referral process in TRICARE is complex because of varying rules applying to its MTF, network, and non-network providers across plans and beneficiaries (GAO, 2019). In the past, TRICARE beneficiaries were required to receive prior authorization and a referral for most specialty care. The MHS has been relaxing these requirements, eliminating the need for a referral for mental health counselors in 2011 and for some urgent care visits starting in 2016 (DHA, 2019). Prior work has found that gatekeeping functions, such as specialty referrals and prior authorizations, reduce patient satisfaction (Kerr et al., 1999). Evidence also indicates that choice of physician is more highly valued among Americans than in other countries (Hero et al., 2016). Therefore, some of the frustration in accessing services could be linked to continued difficulty accessing referrals.

Routine Care

Eighty-seven percent of caregivers of TRICARE-covered children with SHCN reported having a usual place to take their children when they were sick or needed medical advice, rates similar to commercially and publicly insured children (86 percent and 85 percent) but higher than uninsured children (73 percent). We found similar results for having a usual source of preventive care. However, caregivers of TRICARE-covered children with SHCN were less likely than those of commercially or publicly insured children to report having a personal physician or other health care provider (71 percent versus 82 percent and 80 percent, respectively).

Specialist Care

Caregivers of TRICARE-covered children were significantly more likely to report needing a referral to see a doctor than those with children in any other insurance category. Among children with SHCN (who would be more likely to need specialist care), 54 percent of those with TRICARE needed a referral, compared with 31 percent in commercial plans and 42 percent in public plans. Among those children who needed a referral, caregivers of TRICARE-covered children with SHCN were more likely than those of commercially insured children with

SHCN to report that it was somewhat or very difficult to get referrals (32 percent versus 18 percent). However, we did not find evidence that it was any more difficult for TRICARE-covered children with SHCN to receive needed mental health or specialist care than children in any other insurance category.

Getting Needed Care

Six percent of caregivers of TRICARE-covered children with SHCN reported not getting needed health care in the year prior to the survey, similar to rates among children with SHCN in commercial or public insurance plans (4 percent and 6 percent) and significantly lower than uninsured children with SHCN (17 percent).

Care Coordination

Caregivers of TRICARE-covered children with SHCN were more likely than caregivers of the commercially insured children with SHCN to report having someone help with care coordination (32 percent versus 22 percent). However, caregivers of TRICARE-covered children with SHCN were more likely than caregivers of commercially insured children to report feeling like they needed more help coordinating their child's care (22 percent versus 13 percent).

Insurance Coverage and Affordability

Caregivers of TRICARE-covered children with SHCN were less likely to report problems paying for any of their child's medical or health care bills than those in other coverage categories. Twelve percent of caregivers of TRICARE-covered children with SHCN reported problems paying medical bills, compared with 23 percent in the commercially insured, 21 percent in the publicly insured, and 44 percent in the uninsured categories.

Patient Centeredness

Caregivers of TRICARE-covered children reported high degrees of shared decisionmaking. Ninety-two percent of caregivers of TRICARE-covered children with SHCN reported care consistent with a shared decisionmaking model, on par with caregivers of commercially insured children with SHCN and higher than caregivers of publicly insured children and uninsured children (88 percent, 82 percent and 78 percent, respectively). Caregivers of TRICARE-covered children with SHCN reported higher degrees of frustration ("usually" or "always" frustrated) getting services than those of commercially insured children with SHCN (33 percent versus 26 percent) and similar degrees of frustration as those of publicly insured children with SHCN. Caregivers of uninsured children with SHCN reported higher levels of frustration than those in TRICARE, but the difference was not statistically significant.

Summary

Although there is no single definition of SHCN across TRICARE, we used a standardized five-item screening tool developed by the Child and Adolescent Health Measurement Initiative and based on a definition of SHCN developed by the Maternal and Child Health Bureau of the Health Resources and Services Administration to compare TRICARE-covered children with and without SHCN. Roughly 20 percent of TRICARE-covered children in our sample were identified as having SHCN through this screener, which roughly corresponded to the 17 percent of MHS-enrolled children who were found to have a noncomplex chronic condition in 2015 in an analysis of claims.

Caregivers of TRICARE-covered children with SHCN reported more difficulty getting referrals, were less likely to get needed care, had more frustration getting care, and had a greater desire for more help coordinating care compared with caregivers of TRICARE-covered children without SHCN. MFLS respondents with children with SHCN were less likely to report receiving timely care, less likely to report receiving timely pediatric referrals, were less satisfied with ease of access and the quality of their providers overall than respondents without children with SHCN. Caregivers of TRICARE-covered children who had ever had MBHCN reported no difference in accessing routine care compared with those whose children never had MBHCN, but they had more difficulty accessing specialty care, were less likely to receive care for their child when needed, and were more frustrated getting care. They also reported needing more assistance coordinating care and had problems paying for care even though they reported that their insurance covered MBHCN. TRICARE-covered families with *both* SHCN and MBHCN reported substantially worse access experiences than families with just one or neither designation.

Comparing TRICARE-covered children with SHCN and children with SHCN with other or no insurance, we found that caregivers of TRICARE-covered children were more likely to report a usual place of care than those with children on public insurance but were less likely to report having a personal physician or other health care provider than those with children on commercial and public insurance. TRICARE-covered children were more likely to need a referral and had more difficulty getting referrals than their counterparts with other types of insurance. There was no difference between TRICARE-covered children and children with other insurance coverage in terms of receipt of needed mental health or specialist care. Caregivers of TRICARE-covered children were more likely to report having someone to help with care coordination among doctors and services but were also more likely to report feeling like they needed more help coordinating their child's care than those with commercial insurance. Therefore, free programs in TRICARE that assist with care coordination, such as the EFMP or case management services, may not be sufficiently utilized or could fall short of what some military families need. Caregivers of TRICARE-covered children with SHCN were less likely than those with other insurance or no insurance to report problems paying for any of their child's medical or health care bills. Our results of comparable access experiences among children with SHCN in TRICARE relative to other insurance groups contrast with prior research that has shown worse health care access and quality for TRICARE-covered children with SHCN compared with nonmilitary children.

CHAPTER FIVE

Impact of Relocations on Access to Care for TRICARE-Covered Children

For many active-component service members, frequent relocations are considered a part of military life. Active-duty service members in the United States can expect to move with their families to a new station every three years, although many relocate more frequently. Prior research has shown that children who move frequently have less overall access to routine and sick care and are less likely to have a usual source of care than children who move less frequently. These findings have been long-standing: In a study using data from the 1988 wave of the National Health Interview Survey of Child Health, researchers found that children who moved more than three times had less access overall to regular and sick care than those who did not move. Similarly, those who moved at least twice were three times as likely to lack a regular site for preventive or sick care and 1.6 times as likely to use the emergency room as those who never moved (Fowler, Simpson, and Schoendorf, 1993).

An analysis of 2007 NSCH data found that children who moved more than three times were more likely to report poorer overall health, poorer oral health, and one or more chronic conditions. They were also more likely to be uninsured, have gaps in health coverage, and lack a regular site of care (Busacker and Kasehagen, 2012). These factors may be especially problematic for children with SHCN (Newacheck et al., 2000), who need to use the health system more frequently and are already at higher risk of poor access. As with relocations among the civilian population, military relocations disrupt existing relationships with health care providers, place administrative burdens on families, and make it difficult to maintain care continuity.

The challenges for military families that accompany person-nel on service-related relocations are well recognized within DoD. Helping families with the difficulties of relocation is one of the pri-mary roles of the EFMP. The NDAA for FY 2018 required the Sec-retary of Defense to produce a plan to mitigate the impact of PCS and other service-related relocations on the continuity of health care services received by children with special medical or behavioral needs (Pub. L. 115-91, 2017). Part of this plan included developing a col-laborative group of representatives from all service components and programs of the MHS to gather data and monitor the impact of reloca-tions on children with SHCN, with data-gathering scheduled to com-mence in late 2019. However, we were unable to identify recent efforts that characterized or quantified the effects of relocations on families across the TRICARE system.

In this chapter, we compare the access experiences of children who move more frequently with those of children who move less frequently, both among all children and among TRICARE-covered children, to assess the impact that service-related relocation may have on the experiences of military families.

Approach

To explore the role of relocations in health care access experiences, we used the NSCH to examine pediatric access outcomes by rate of address changes over the course of a child's life. We wanted to examine whether the rate of address changes was associated with negative access experiences across the broader population of children and among children with SHCN, as well as the impact of address changes among TRICARE-covered children, in particular, in terms of caregiver-reported access challenges. We began by looking at the impact of frequent address changes among all children in the sample by SHCN status and then focused on the impact of frequent address changes for children covered by TRICARE. We categorized children into three levels of relocation frequency: (1) no moves in their lifetime; (2) at least one move but less than one move every two years; and (3) at least one move every two years. The first and third categories correspond to roughly the bottom and top fifth of the distribution of address-change frequency among TRICARE-covered children and allowed us to detect an impact of address changes that affected a large portion of the TRICARE-covered population. We compared the bottom category to the other two categories by SHCN status using multivariable logistic regression, adjusting for sociodemographics, such as insurance status (described in more detail in Chapter Two), and including an interaction between address change frequency and SHCN status. We used these models to estimate the average predicted probabilities for each category of move frequency. For the within-TRICARE analysis, due to sample-size constraints, we estimated our models while adjusting only for survey years. We calculated rate of address changes by dividing the number of reported address changes by the child's age.

We then used MFLS data to compare reported access and quality of care before and after PCS for all TRICARE-covered children. We then used multivariable logistic regression with sociodemographic controls (described in more detail in Chapter Two) to compare the average marginal effects of TRICARE insurance type and service branch on access and quality disruptions due to PCS.

Limitations

Our measure of frequency of address changes does not account for average distance moved and therefore may not capture all the elements that could make a move disruptive to health care. Address changes among TRICARE enrollees due to service-related relocations are likely moves of longer distance and may be more disruptive than those among the civilian population. Because of sample-size constraints, we were not able to assess the impact of relocations on TRICARE-covered children with SHCN separately from the rest of the survey sample of children with SHCN, so our results may underestimate the impacts of relocation on health care for these military children. In addition, service members enrolled in TRICARE might choose not to move their families when they are relocated to avoid disruptions to education and health care. Differences in access experiences between families that move frequently and those that do not could therefore partially reflect underlying differences in TRICARE service members who move their families for PCS and those who do not.

Results

The NSCH data analysis confirmed that TRICARE-covered children experience more address changes in their lives than children in other insurance categories. Twenty-one percent of TRICARE-covered children were reported to have moved more than once every two years of their lives, compared with 15 percent of children on public insurance and only 6 percent of commercially insured children (Table 5.1).

Impact of Address Changes on Access

Across insurance categories, caregivers of children with and without SHCN who frequently changed their home address reported worse access to pediatric care in several domains compared with caregivers

Table 5.1
Rate of Address Changes, by Insurance Type

Insurance Type	Rate of Address Change (%)		
	No Moves	At Least 1 Move, Less than 1 Every 2 Years	More Than Once Every 2 Years
Number in sample	35,696	52,462	7,374
TRICARE	18	61	21
Commercial	40	54	6
Public	27	58	15
None	33	57	11
Other	32	59	10

SOURCE: Analysis of 2016–2018 NSCH data, weighted for survey design.
NOTE: Pearson chi-squared test $p < 0.0001$.

who had not moved during the child's life. Among families with children with SHCN, there were few differences by address change frequency in having a usual source of routine preventive care or care when the child was sick; however, there were significant differences in access experiences related to specialty care (Table 5.2). Compared with caregivers of children with SHCN who had not moved, caregivers of children with SHCN who had moved at least once every two years ("frequent movers") reported greater difficulty getting a referral (31 percent versus 21 percent), were more likely to report difficulty getting mental health treatment (59 percent versus 46 percent), and were more likely to report difficulty getting specialist care (34 verses 25 percent) for their children. Frequent movers were more likely than never-movers to not get the care their children needed (9 percent versus 5 percent). Frequent movers were also more likely to report difficulty paying medical bills (30 versus 23 percent) and more likely to report frustration getting care (40 versus 30 percent).

These patterns were largely the same for children without SHCN. In this group, frequent movers were less likely than caregivers of children who never moved to have one or more people they considered to be their child's doctor or nurse, perhaps reflecting a lower need for care causing a longer disruption in having a regular caregiver after a move.

Across all TRICARE respondents, frequent movers were more likely to report difficulty getting a referral than never-movers (34 percent versus 16 percent), higher degrees of frustration getting services (22 percent versus 13 percent), and needing additional help coordinating their child's care (16 percent versus 6 percent) (Table 5.3). The large difference in a desire for more care coordination was notable, given the lack of such an association in the general population.

We used the MFLS data to investigate differential effects of PCS across TRICARE plan type and service branch. Caregivers with children in TRICARE Select were, on average, 6.7 percentage points less likely to agree that they could access the same quality of pediatric care for their child after PCS (Table 5.4). This result indicates that service members with TRICARE Select, whose reliance on network care may equate to less consistency in access and quality across the country,

Table 5.2
Pediatric Access Experiences Among Children, by Rate of Address Changes over Child's Life and SHCN Status

Access Category	SHCN (%)			No SHCN (%)		
	No Moves	At Least 1 Move, Less Than 1 Every 2 Years	More Than 1 Move Every 2 Years	No Moves	At Least 1 Move, Less Than 1 Every 2 Years	More Than 1 Move Every 2 Years
Number in sample	6,741	13,613	1,979	28,955	38,813	5,395
Usual source of care						
Has usual source of care when child is sick	87	84	84	79	78	77
Has usual source of care for child's routine preventive care	95	95	95	92	92	91
Caregiver thinks of one or more persons as child's doctor or nurse	83	79*	81	73	71**	68***
Specialist care (in past year)						
Child needed referral	37	34	45**	13	13	14
Had difficulty getting a referral	21	23	31**	14	18*	22**
Had difficulty getting mental health treatment	46	45	59**	40	37	43
Had difficulty getting specialist care	25	28	34*	20	23	31**
Getting needed care (in past year)						
Child needed care but did not receive it	5	6	9*	1	2***	4***

Table 5.2—Continued

Access Category	SHCN (%)			No SHCN (%)		
	No Moves	At Least 1 Move, Less Than 1 Every 2 Years	More Than 1 Move Every 2 Years	No Moves	At Least 1 Move, Less Than 1 Every 2 Years	More Than 1 Move Every 2 Years
Care coordination (in past year)						
Received help coordinating care	24	24	26	16	16	15
Could have used more help coordinating care	15	13	18	4	4	7***
Insurance coverage and affordability						
Health insurance usually covers child's health care needs	90	91	91	95	94	94*
Health insurance usually allows child to see health care provider	94	95	94	97	97*	96**
Health insurance usually covers child's MBHCN	73	74	76	72	68	68
Had problems paying health care bills in past year	23	23	30*	12	14	15*
Patient-centeredness (in past year)						
Usually frustrated getting health care services	30	29	40***	11	14***	18***
Health care providers usually responsive to concerns	85	86	84	89	85*	89

SOURCE: Analysis of 2016–2018 NSCH data.

NOTES: All percentages represent average predicted probabilities, adjusted for sociodemographics. Tests of significance performed using Wald tests of coefficients relative to the reference category. In 64 tests, we would expect 2.6 significant results due to chance alone at $p < 0.05$, 0.6 significant results at $p < 0.01$, and 0.06 significant results at $p < 0.001$, assuming all tests are independent.
* $p < 0.05$, ** $p < 0.01$, *** $p < 0.001$.

Table 5.3
Pediatric Access Experiences Among All TRICARE-Covered Children, by Rate of Address Changes over Child's Life

Access Category	Rate of Address Change (%)		
	Never Moved	At Least 1 Move, Less Than 1 Every 2 Years	More Than 1 Move Every 2 Years
Number in sample	560	1,951	561
Usual source of care			
Has usual source of care when child is sick	86	84	78
Has usual source of care for child's routine preventive care	97	96	95
Caregiver thinks of one or more persons as child's doctor or nurse	73	71	67
Specialist care (in past year)			
Child needed referral	25	28	25
Had difficulty getting a referral	16	28	34*
Had difficulty getting mental health treatment	46	45	49
Had difficulty getting specialist care	22	25	39
Getting needed care (in past year)			
Child needed care but did not receive it	2	3	4
Care coordination (in past year)			
Received help coordinating care	32	26	21
Could have used more help coordinating care in last year	6	8	16*
Insurance coverage and affordability			
Health insurance usually covers child's health needs	97	94	96
Health insurance usually allows child to see health care provider	97	97	93

Table 5.3—Continued

Access Category	Rate of Address Change (%)		
	Never Moved	At Least 1 Move, Less Than 1 Every 2 Years	More Than 1 Move Every 2 Years
Health insurance usually covers child's MBHCN	88	79	82
Had problems paying for health care bills	12	12	14
Patient-centeredness (in past year)			
Usually frustrated getting health care services	13	20*	22*
Health care providers usually responsive to concerns	89	91	87

SOURCE: Analysis of 2016–2018 NSCH data.

NOTES: All percentages represent average predicted probabilities, adjusted for sociodemographics. Tests of significance performed using Wald tests of coefficients relative to the reference category. In 32 tests, we would expect 1.6 significant results due to chance alone at $p < 0.05$, assuming all tests are independent.
* $p < 0.05$.

Table 5.4
Average Marginal Effects of TRICARE Insurance Type Compared with TRICARE Prime at an MTF

Access Category	TRICARE Plan/Care Setting (%)		
	TRICARE Prime (PCM at MTF)	TRICARE Prime (Network PCM)	TRICARE Select
Number in sample	2,067	1,003	553
Able to access and continue same quality of pediatric care after PCS (60% agree overall)	(Reference)	+0.0	−6.7*

SOURCE: Analysis of MFLS data.

NOTES: Table shows average marginal effects of different insurance categories relative to the reference. Numbers express, on average, how much more or less likely an individual in the sample would be to give the response if they were recategorized from the reference category to the new category. In two tests, we would expect less than one significant result due to chance alone at $p < 0.05$, assuming all tests are independent. * $p < 0.05$.

may be particularly vulnerable to care disruption after a move. No statistically significant differences were observed across service branches (Table 5.5).

Across our analyses, we found evidence that frequent moves in the TRICARE population presented a significant barrier to accessing care and may have contributed to the frustration that TRICARE caregivers reported in accessing services, consistent with prior research (Aronson et al., 2016; Fowler, Simpson, and Schoendorf, 1993; Jelleyman and Spencer, 2008). Differences between TRICARE-covered families and the general population in the access barriers associated with frequent moving may be instructive. In the general population, frequent movers were more likely than never-movers to report not getting needed care or having trouble paying health care bills, which may be expected if disruptions in insurance coverage or access to covered providers coincides with a change of address. For TRICARE enrollees, for whom insurance-related disruptions would not occur with relocation, we observed no such associations between frequent moves and accessing needed care or paying for care. In TRICARE, frequent moves were more strongly associated with administrative challenges, including difficulty getting a referral, frustration getting care, and a desire for more assistance with care coordination. We did not find

Table 5.5
Average Marginal Effects of Military Service Branch Compared with Army

	Military Service Branch (%)			
Access Category	Army	Navy	Air Force	Marine Corps
Number in sample	1,383	866	948	533
Able to access and continue same quality of pediatric care after PCS (60% agree overall)	(Reference)	+3.8	−3.6	−1.0

SOURCE: Analysis of MFLS data.

NOTES: Table shows average marginal effects of different insurance categories relative to the reference. Numbers express, on average, how much more or less likely an individual in the sample would be to give the response if they were recategorized from the reference category to the new category.

a strong positive relationship between frequent address changes and a desire for more assistance with care coordination among children with SHCN overall, suggesting that the challenges that TRICARE families face in managing children's complex health care needs may be greatest after relocation.

Summary

Previous literature has found a negative impact from frequent changes of address on pediatric care access and continuity. These disruptions may be particularly detrimental to families with children with SHCN, who use the health care system more frequently and benefit from providers who are familiar with their medical histories. Changing address every few years is a way of life for many service members and their families, and it could affect their experiences accessing pediatric care across the TRICARE system. Programs and policies are in place within DoD to help military families with these transitions, but availability, use, and access to those services varies. Therefore, we examined the impact of frequent change of address on access experiences in our sample overall, stratifying by SHCN status. We also examined the impact of address-change frequency on access experiences within TRICARE and the impact of PCS on care continuity. We categorized children into three levels of relocation frequency: (1) no moves in lifetime, (2) at least one move but less than one move every two years, and (3) at least one move every two years.

NSCH data confirmed that TRICARE-covered children experienced more address changes in their lives than children with other types of insurance. For children with SHCN, overall, caregivers of those who had frequent address changes had greater difficulty getting a referral, were more likely to report difficulty getting mental health treatment, and were more likely to report difficulty getting specialist care. These caregivers were more likely to report that their children did not get the care they needed, reported more problems paying medical bills, and experienced greater frustration getting services. Among the TRICARE population, families who moved frequently reported significantly higher degrees of forgone care, difficulty getting a referral, frustration getting needed services, and a desire for more care coordination than those who had never moved over a child's life. Caregivers of children with TRICARE Select coverage were less likely than those of children with TRICARE Prime to agree that they could access the same quality of pediatric care for their child after PCS. There were no significant differences in the impact of PCS on care continuity by service branch.

CHAPTER SIX

Summary and Recommendations

This report evaluated the pediatric access experiences of military families enrolled in TRICARE using data from two external data sources: the 2016–2018 NSCH and the 2018 Blue Star Families' MFLS.

We found that, in the years 2016–2018, caregivers of TRICARE-covered children, both overall and with SHCN, reported similar levels of difficulty accessing routine and necessary care as those with commercial and public insurance, while caregivers of uninsured children reported higher levels of difficulty. We also found significantly lower financial barriers to access among the TRICARE-insured than in all other coverage groups, likely reflecting the low cost-sharing in TRICARE plans relative to most other types of insurance. Areas of access in which TRICARE underperformed relative to other insurance types included having an individual who was considered the child's personal doctor or nurse, obtaining referrals for needed care, and frustration in getting needed services.

Among children with TRICARE coverage and across TRICARE plans, we identified several areas of vulnerability. Caregivers of TRICARE-covered children with SHCN and MBHCN reported worse access experiences than those whose children did not have special needs, especially in terms of receiving specialist care, getting needed care, and getting assistance with care coordination. We also found evidence that PCS and other service-related relocations are disruptive to pediatric care access, particularly in the areas of obtaining needed referrals and frustration in obtaining needed services. Caregivers of

TRICARE-covered children who changed address frequently were roughly twice as likely to desire more assistance coordinating care than those who had never moved over a child's life. Data from MFLS respondents suggested that the difficulties associated with PCS may be more pronounced among TRICARE Select enrollees than among those with TRICARE Prime. However, data from the same source also indicated caregivers of children with TRICARE Prime with a network PCM and those with TRICARE Select were the most likely to agree that these children received timely pediatric care when it was needed and were more satisfied with the overall ease of access and timeliness of their children's health care. These rates were lower for Air Force children, however. Their caregivers reported greater difficulty obtaining timely referrals and were less satisfied with the quality of providers.

Finally, we found that, among children with TRICARE coverage, those from active-duty families were less likely than children from non–active-duty families to have difficulty obtaining health care (including mental and behavioral health care), and their families were less likely to report trouble paying medical bills. Active-duty families were also less likely to report not getting needed care.

Recommendations

Routinely Collect Pediatric Patient Experience Data

Currently, external sources of data are the only means of comprehensively tracking the health care experiences of the entire population of TRICARE-covered children and assessing those experiences against civilian benchmarks. Although there have been several internal MHS surveys of patient experiences, they have been variably compromised by low response rates and population exclusions that limited their representativeness and their comparability with data on other health systems.

Recent reforms, including the FY 2017 NDAA, included sweeping changes to the organization and administration of the MHS that may improve the ability to track pediatric access and quality, including a reduction in the number of administrative regions and the central-ization of administration and management of MTFs. These reforms could mitigate some of the issues identified in this report, such as access disruptions caused by PCS, by reducing the administrative burdens of transitions and standardizing the records necessary to track access and quality (Pub. L. 115-91, 2017). However, there is no mechanism for MHS-wide tracking of pediatric access and quality of care *experiences*, limiting the ability to assess how these changes may be affect-ing beneficiaries (DHB, 2017). External data sources, such as those used in our study, could help fill the gap, but detailed evaluations of the determinants of pediatric health care experiences, how they vary across the MHS, and how they compare with external benchmarks will require more-targeted data collection, such as through a periodic survey of pediatric access and quality using standard metrics designed for comparison across health systems.

In the past, DHA collected standardized measures of the health care experiences of TRICARE-covered children under age 18 through the HCSDB, but the child survey has not been fielded since 2010 (reflecting 2009 data) (TRICARE, 2009). Unlike current surveys of experiences, the HCSDB child survey collected data on the entire population of DoD beneficiaries, and response rates were generally above 20 percent (Mathematica Policy Research, 2010). Restarting data collection would better position DHA to adopt a more patient-centered orientation as recommended by the DHB in its 2017 evaluation of pediatric care in the MHS, and it would permit an evaluation of how program reforms have affected the experiences of TRICARE members. Ongoing collection of systemwide metrics of pediatric experience would provide a needed guide for the development and adjustment of ongoing quality improvement efforts by identifying areas where the system is deficient or does not meet patient expectations. Such systematic data collection would also provide DHA with the flexibility—through the addition of questions on an as-needed basis—to further evaluate potentially problematic areas of patient care, such the availability and sufficiency of care coordination for children with SHCN. Finally, the standardized measures in the HCSDB would also enable ongoing comparisons of pediatric access and quality between

TRICARE enrollees and civilian populations, a role currently filled through analyses of secondary data that may suffer from issues of misclassification and lack of representativeness.

Further Streamline Referrals and Monitor Effects on Patient Experience Through Improved Data Collection

Our analysis of NSCH data indicates that the referral process was a source of difficulty for TRICARE beneficiaries accessing pediatric care in the 2016–2018 period. This was especially true for children with SHCN. These findings lend support to changes initiated by the MHS in 2017 to streamline and expedite the referral process through improved data collection and policies (DHB, 2017). Among these changes is the ability to separately track the time between referral and booking and the time between booking and appointment, enabling more-consistent measurement of referral times across the MHS, something that has been reported since FY 2019.

The MHS also recently implemented other changes that could reduce difficulty of obtaining specialty referrals for patients and providers. Referral requirements have been relaxed or eliminated for several types of care, including urgent and preventive care (DHA, 2019). Additionally, over the 2017–2018 period, specialty referral guidance was developed and standardized across the MHS to facilitate referrals both within the direct care system and between direct and network care providers (GAO, 2019; MHS, 2017). The effects of these changes would not have been captured in the data that we analyzed. Future years of NSCH data could provide insight into whether these initiatives have improved the perceived ease of getting a referral among the TRICARE population overall; however, an evaluation with actionable results would require data capturing variation across the MHS. The requirements for referrals differ by TRICARE plan, locus of referral, and other factors, and further information on how patient experiences vary would greatly improve understanding of the role of referrals.

Fully Implement DoD Plans to Monitor Effects of Permanent Change of Station and Other Service-Related Relocations

Our findings indicate that frequent relocations exacerbate the difficulties and frustrations that families with TRICARE-covered children with SHCN face when navigating a health system that can be complex and administratively burdensome (Aronson et al., 2016). Recent legislation required DoD to produce a plan to mitigate the impact of relocations on military children with SHCN (Pub. L. 115-91, 2017). In response, DoD developed a collaborative group representing all components and MHS programs to gather data and monitor the effects of relocations on children with SHCN, and data gathering was scheduled to commence in late 2019 (DoD, 2018a).

Our results suggest that this effort should include measures of beneficiary experiences accessing care to identify specific family circumstances—such as the type and severity of a child's health needs or use of available programs and resources—that lead to or mitigate caregiver frustrations after a move. For instance, service members with children with special needs are eligible to enroll in the EFMP, which ensures that special needs are considered during relocations and provides assistance connecting service members to available resources and benefits when they are assigned to a new location. Unfortunately, the type and degree of assistance available through the EFMP has reportedly been uneven across locations and service branches (DHB, 2017).

In 2018, GAO reviewed EFMP services and recommended that DoD produce a common set of metrics and monitoring standards to evaluate the assignment coordination and family support provided through the program. DoD signaled that it planned to follow these recommendations (GAO, 2018). As part of a set of common metrics of EFMP performance, patient experience data collected from recently relocated families, combined with administrative data on program and resource use, could be used to identify variations in program effectiveness.

Review the Availability and Use of Care Coordination Services for Children with Complex Health Conditions

Many caregivers of TRICARE-covered children with SHCN reported wanting more assistance coordinating their child's health care, despite being more likely to report receiving care coordination assistance than caregivers of other insured children. The MHS provides access to care coordination through several mechanisms. TRICARE members with complex health conditions may be eligible for case management services at no cost (TRICARE, 2019). In 2009, the MHS established the Patient Centered Medical Home as its primary care model, which encourages coordination and integration through team-based care led by a PCM. Additionally, PCMs and 24-hour helplines operated by Military OneSource and the MHS Nurse Advice Line may fulfill limited coordination and assistance roles (TRICARE, 2019). However, unreliable documentation has made it difficult to track and evaluate utilization rates and the effectiveness of TRICARE case management services. For instance, a 2013 DoD review of case management enrollment among TRICARE members with serious mental health issues drew few conclusions due to insufficient data quality (DoD, TRICARE Management Activity, 2013).

Our results suggest that, as of the 2016–2018 period, a significant degree of demand for assistance in coordinating care for TRICARE-covered children with SHCN was unmet. Better access to more-effective care coordination might improve experiences where they fell short of other insurance groups, including difficulty with the referral process and frustration in obtaining needed services. The MHS is well positioned through its PCM model to improve and expand the coordination services it provides. A broad review of the availability, source, and use of care coordination for children with SHCN could help identify promising approaches for achieving this goal.

Areas for Further Investigation

Our research highlighted a need for additional study in several areas:

- MFLS data indicate that the access experiences of caregivers of TRICARE-covered children may vary by service branch. MTFs have traditionally been staffed and managed by the medical departments of the service branches. Differences in how the services manage care for dependents under age 18 and the possible implications for health care experiences should be investigated. The process to transition administration and management of the MTFs to the DHA began in October 2018, with direct support still coming from the services' medical departments (Donovan, 2019). This effort, which has a primary goal of improving force readiness through greater centralization, is resulting in a major reorganization of the MHS with possible implications for dependent care. Therefore, it will be important to monitor what impact the transition may have on pediatric access across the service branches.

- MFLS data showed evidence of variation in experiences of care timeliness by geographic location. Concerns about the adequacy of the civilian provider network in rural and other underserved areas have been raised at various points. TRICARE is required to submit network adequacy reports to monitor whether member access needs are being met (Backhus, 2000; Kanof, 2003). However, prior evaluations found that these reports were insufficient to measure adequacy, given that they indicate only whether providers are in-network, not whether they are accepting new patients. To investigate these issues, the MHS could cross-reference its provider files (network and MTF) with utilization records and pediatric specialty care availability to determine provider density by geographic area.

- Evidence of significant disruptions in care access and continuity due to service-related relocations indicates a need to evaluate the programs in place to assist families during these transitions, such as the EFMP. Our results suggest that frustrations with accessing care and a desire for more care coordination are a system-wide issue for caregivers of TRICARE-covered children who move frequently—and not just among those with children with SHCN. Therefore, future investigations should also consider whether transitional assistance during relocations should be made available to a wider set of families than those that are currently eligible.

Detailed Analytic Results

This appendix provides additional detail on our analytic results. Figure A.1 shows the geographic representation of respondents to

Figure A.1
Geographic Representativeness of the 2018 Military Family Life Survey Sample

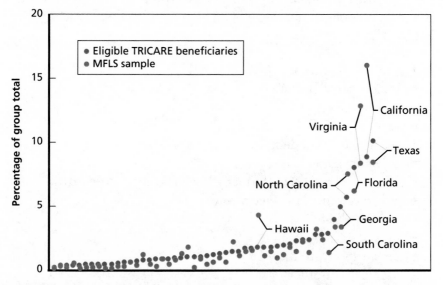

SOURCE: Analysis of 2018 MFLS and state-level enrollment data from MHS administrative data systems as of the end of FY 2018 (DHA, 2019).

NOTE: States are organized in order from smallest to largest percentage of total enrolled MHS population. Labeled states are those whose sample representation differs the most from MHS administrative data.

the 2018 MFLS, conducted by Blue Star Families, compared with the states where MHS beneficiaries reside.

Table A.1 includes the primary access categories used in our analysis of NSCH data, along with descriptions of changes in question wording or response options between the 2016 and 2017 survey waves and the 2018 survey wave. Most categories showed no change, but a few had modifications to either the question or the response options.

Table A.2 shows the number of observations in the 2018 MFLS by TRICARE plan type. The most common were TRICARE Prime with a PCM at an MTF and TRICARE Prime with a network PCM, while the least common were TRICARE Select Overseas and TRICARE Retired Reserve.

Table A.3 shows the number of observations in the 2018 MFLS by service. The largest numbers of observations were for the Army and Air Force, and the fewest were for the Coast Guard and U.S. Public Health Service.

We used the following mental, behavioral, and developmental health conditions from the NSCH to identify children with prior MBHCN:

- Tourette syndrome
- anxiety problems
- depression
- substance use disorder
- behavioral or conduct problems
- developmental delay
- intellectual disability (formerly known as mental retardation)
- speech or other language disorder
- learning disability
- autism
- autism spectrum disorder
- Asperger's disorder
- pervasive developmental disorder
- attention deficit disorder
- attention-deficit/hyperactivity disorder.

Table A.1
National Survey of Children's Health Year-to-Year Question Wording and Other Changes

Access Characteristic	Type of Change	2016 and 2017 Version	2018 Version	Positive Response Specification and Reference Group
Usual source of care (sick)	Change in question	Is there a place that this child USUALLY goes when he or she is sick or you or another caregiver needs advice about his or her health?	Is there a place you or another caregiver USUALLY take this child when he or she is sick, or you need advice about his or her health?	Yes No (reference)
Usual source of care (well)	No change	Is there a place that this child USUALLY goes when he or she needs routine preventive care, such as a physical examination or well-child check-up?		Yes No (reference)
Personal doctor	No change	Do you have one or more persons you think of as this child's personal doctor or nurse? A personal doctor or nurse is a health professional who knows this child well and is familiar with this child's health history. This can be a general doctor, a pediatrician, a specialist doctor, a nurse practitioner, or a physician's assistant.		Yes, one person OR Yes, more than one person No (reference)
Need for a referral	No change	DURING THE PAST 12 MONTHS, did this child need a referral to see any doctors or receive any services?		Yes No (reference)
Problem getting a referral	Change in question and response options	How much of a problem was it to get referrals? 1 = Not a problem 2 = Small problem 3 = Big problem	How difficult was it to get referrals? 1 = Not difficult 2 = Somewhat difficult 3 = Very difficult 4 = It was not possible to get a referral	Small problem OR big problem OR somewhat difficult OR very difficult OR It was not possible to get a referral Not a problem OR Not difficult (reference)

Table A.1—Continued

Access Characteristic	Type of Change	2016 and 2017 Version	2018 Version	Positive Response Specification and Reference Group
Problem getting mental health treatment	Change in question and response options	How much of a problem was it to get the mental health treatment or counseling that this child needed? 1 = Not a problem 2 = Small problem 3 = Big problem	How difficult was it to get the mental health treatment or counseling that this child needed? 1 = Not difficult 2 = Somewhat difficult 3 = Very difficult 4 = It was not possible to get a referral	Small problem OR big problem OR somewhat difficult OR very difficult OR It was not possible to get a referral Not a problem OR not difficult (reference)
Problem getting specialist care	Change in question and response options	How much of a problem was it to get the specialist care that this child needed? 1 = Not a problem 2 = Small problem 3 = Big problem	How difficult was it to get the specialist care that this child needed? 1 = Not difficult 2 = Somewhat difficult 3 = Very difficult 4 = It was not possible to get a referral	Small problem OR big problem OR somewhat difficult OR very difficult OR It was not possible to get a referral Not a problem OR not difficult (reference)
Getting needed care	No change	DURING THE PAST 12 MONTHS, was there any time when this child needed health care, but it was not received? By health care, we mean medical care as well as other kinds of care like dental care, vision care, and mental health services.		Yes No (reference)
Coordination of child's care	Change in question	Does anyone help you arrange or coordinate this child's care among the different doctors or services that this child uses?	DURING THE PAST 12 MONTHS, did anyone help you arrange or coordinate this child's care among the different doctors or services that this child uses?	Yes; No OR did not see more than one health care provider in past 12 months (reference)

Table A.1—Continued

Access Characteristic	Type of Change	2016 and 2017 Version	2018 Version	Positive Response Specification and Reference Group
Extra help coordinating care	No change	DURING THE PAST 12 MONTHS, have you felt that you could have used extra help arranging or coordinating this child's care among the different health care providers or services?	Yes; No (reference)	Extra help coordinating care
Insurance coverage: adequate benefits	No change	How often does this child's health insurance offer benefits or cover services that meet this child's needs?		Usually OR always Sometime OR never (reference)
Insurance coverage: see needed providers	No change	How often does this child's health insurance allow him or her to see the health care providers he or she needs?		Usually OR always Sometimes OR never (reference)
Insurance coverage: mental or behavioral needs	No change	Thinking specifically about this child's mental or behavioral health needs, how often does this child's health insurance offer benefits or cover services that meet these needs?		Usually OR always Sometime OR never (reference)
Insurance coverage: problems paying	No change	DURING THE PAST 12 MONTHS, did your family have problems paying for any of this child's medical or health care bills?		Yes No (reference)

Table A.1—Continued

Access Characteristic	Type of Change	2016 and 2017 Version	2018 Version	Positive Response Specification and Reference Group
Family-centered care/shared decisionmaking	No change	[Only asked of parents who indicated that the child needed decisions to be made regarding their health care.] DURING THE PAST 12 MONTHS, how often did this child's doctors or other health care providers: Discuss with you the range of options to consider for his or her health care or treatment? Work with you to decide together which health care and treatment choices would be best for this child? Make it easy for you to raise concerns or disagree with recommendations for this child's health care?	Usually OR always Sometime OR never (reference)
Frustrated getting care	No change	DURING THE PAST 12 MONTHS, how often were you frustrated in your efforts to get services for this child?		Sometimes OR usually OR always Never (reference)

Table A.2
Number of Observations, by TRICARE Insurance Type,
Military Family Life Survey

TRICARE Insurance Type	Number Reporting Coverage
TRICARE Prime (PCM at MTF)	2,067
TRICARE Prime (network PCM)	786
TRICARE Remote	130
TRICARE Overseas	105
TRICARE Remote Overseas	13
TRICARE Select	553
TRICARE Select Overseas	5
TRICARE for Life	43
TRICARE Reserve Select	118
TRICARE Retired Reserve	8
US Family Health Plan	87

SOURCE: Analysis of 2018 MFLS data.

Table A.3
Number of Observations, by Military Service Branch,
Military Family Life Survey

Military Service Branch	Number in Sample
Army	1,383
Navy	866
Air Force	948
Marine Corps	533
Coast Guard	158
Public Health Service	23

SOURCE: Analysis of 2018 MFLS data.

In addition to these conditions, children were also designated as having MBHCN if caregivers reported that a doctor or other health care provider had ever told them that their child had "any other mental health condition."

Table A.4 shows the pooled percentage of observations in the NSCH data for each access category by SHCN and MBHCN. TRICARE-covered families with *both* SHCN and MBHCN reported substantially worse access experiences than those with neither type of need, including difficulty getting a referral, difficulty getting specialist care, not getting needed care, and frustration getting care. They were also significantly more likely to report that they could have used more help coordinating care and less likely to say that their plan usually allowed them to see the doctor they wanted.

Tables A.5 and A.6 show robustness checks of the results from Tables 3.2 and 4.4, respectively. These tables use data from caregivers who indicated only one insurance type and exclude those who selected multiple types of insurance.

Table A.4
Pediatric Access Experiences Among TRICARE-Covered Children, by SHCN and MBHCN Status

Access Category	No SHCN (%)		SHCN (%)	
	No MBHCN (reference)	MBHCN	No MBHCN	MBHCN
Number in sample	2,265	251	319	485
Usual source of care				
Has usual source of care when child is sick	81	80	89	88
Has usual source of care for child's routine preventive care	95	95	97	97
Caregiver thinks of one or more persons as child's doctor or nurse	67	74	71	71
Specialist care (in past year)				
Child needed referral	20	31*	46***	54***
Had difficulty getting a referral	19	22	39*	44**

Table A.4—Continued

Access Category	No SHCN (%)		SHCN (%)	
	No MBHCN (reference)	**MBHCN**	**No MBHCN**	**MBHCN**
Had difficulty getting mental health treatment	—	56	—	48
Had difficulty getting specialist care	16	33	26	45**
Getting needed care (in past year)				
Child needed care but did not receive it	2	2	6	9**
Care coordination (in past year)				
Received help coordinating care	23	21	36	30
Could have used more help coordinating care	4	5	11	30***
Insurance coverage and affordability				
Health insurance usually covers child's health needs	95	95	95	90*
Health insurance usually allows child to see health care provider	98	97	98	86***
Health insurance usually covers child's MBHCN	63	90*	94*	86*
Had problems paying health care bills in past year	12	15	11	17
Patient-centeredness (in past year)				
Usually frustrated getting health care services	11	27**	24**	43***
Health care providers usually responsive to concerns	90	84	93	92

SOURCE: Analysis of 2016–2018 NSCH.

NOTES: All percentages represent the average predicted probabilities, adjusted for sociodemographics. For consistency with other studies (e.g., Seshadri, 2019), we report results by MBHCN only for children age 6 and older. Tests of significance performed using Wald tests of coefficients relative to the reference category. In 48 tests, we would expect two significant results due to chance alone at $p < 0.05$, 0.5 significant results at $p < 0.01$, and 0.05 significant results at $p < 0.001$, assuming all tests are independent. * $p < 0.05$, ** $p < 0.01$, *** $p < 0.001$.

Point estimates are largely similar to those in Tables 3.2 and 4.4. However, due to smaller sample sizes, some of the results are statistically weaker. A notable exception is getting needed care in the past year: Caregivers of TRICARE-covered children were more likely to report not receiving needed care than caregivers of commercially insured children (5 percent versus 3 percent across all children; 13 percent versus 5 percent among children with SHCN).

Table A.5
Pediatric Access Experiences, by Insurance Type (alternative parameterization)

Access Category	Insurance Type (%)			
	TRICARE (reference)	Commercial	Public	None
Number in sample	1,281	68,663	18,702	3,632
Usual source of care				
Has usual source of care when child is sick	84	83	77**	63***
Has usual source of care for child's routine preventive care	95	95	92	74***
Caregiver thinks of one or more persons as child's doctor or nurse	72	77	71	52***
Specialist care (in past year)				
Child needed referral	29	16***	20***	14***
Had difficulty getting a referral	30	15**	24	36
Had difficulty getting mental health treatment	49	46	41	52
Had difficulty getting specialist care	27	21	29	34
Getting needed care (in past year)				
Child needed care but did not receive it	5	2**	3	10
Care coordination (in past year)				
Received help coordinating care	24	17*	20	15*

Table A.5—Continued

Access Category	Insurance Type (%)			
	TRICARE (reference)	Commercial	Public	None
Could have used more help coordinating care	9	6	9	7
Insurance coverage and affordability				
Health insurance usually covers child's health needs	94	92	96	—
Health insurance usually allows child to see health care provider	96	96	97	—
Health insurance usually covers child's MBHCN	85	66***	78	—
Had problems paying health care bills in past year	6	14***	14***	24***
Patient-centeredness (in past year)				
Usually frustrated getting health care services	18	13**	20	28**
Health care providers usually responsive to concerns	94	89*	83***	81***

SOURCE: Analysis of 2016–2018 NSCH data.

NOTES: All percentages represent average predicted probabilities, adjusted for sociodemographics. Tests of significance performed using Wald tests of coefficients relative to the reference category. In 61 tests, we would expect three significant results due to chance alone at $p < 0.05$, 0.6 significant results at $p < 0.01$, and 0.06 significant results at $p < 0.001$, assuming all tests are independent. * $p < 0.05$, ** $p < 0.01$, *** $p < 0.001$.

Table A.6
Pediatric Access Experiences, by Insurance Type, Among Children with Special Health Care Needs (alternative parameterization)

Access Category	Insurance Type (%)			
	TRICARE (reference)	Commercial	Public	None
Number in sample	227	13,586	5,705	680
Usual source of care				
Has usual source of care when child is sick	87	88	83	71*
Has usual source of care for child's routine preventive care	95	96	95	86
Caregiver thinks of one or more persons as child's doctor or nurse	72	83	79	64
Specialist care (in past year)				
Child needed referral	64	33***	42***	38***
Had difficulty getting a referral	34	19	29	47
Had difficulty getting mental health treatment	52	51	46	54
Had difficulty getting specialist care	25	26	33	42
Getting needed care (in past year)				
Child needed care but was not received	13	5*	8	24
Care coordination (in past year)				
Received help coordinating care	25	22	29	31
Could have used more help coordinating care	20	15	20	18
Insurance coverage and affordability				
Health insurance usually covers child's health needs	90	87	93	—
Health insurance usually allows child to see health care provider	91	93	95	—

Table A.6—Continued

Access Category	Insurance Type (%)			
	TRICARE (reference)	Commercial	Public	None
Health insurance usually covers child's MBHCN	90	69***	85	—
Had problems paying health care bills in past year	15	26	22	49***
Patient-centeredness (in past year)				
Usually frustrated getting health care services	35	29	39	49
Health care providers usually responsive to concerns	96	88**	80***	75***

SOURCE: Analysis of 2016–2018 NSCH data.

NOTES: All percentages represent the average predicted probabilities, adjusted for sociodemographics. Tests of significance performed using Wald tests of coefficients relative to the reference category. In 61 tests, we would expect three significant results due to chance alone at $p < 0.05$, 0.6 significant results at $p < 0.01$ and 0.06 significant results at $p < 0.001$, assuming all tests are independent. * $p < 0.05$, ** $p < 0.01$, *** $p < 0.001$.

References

Adirim, Terry, Elizabeth Hisle-Gorman, and David A. Klein, "Families Covered by TRICARE," *Health Affairs*, Vol. 38, No. 11, November 2019, p. 1951.

Agency for Healthcare Research and Quality, *CAHPS Health Plan Survey and Reporting Kit 2008: About the Item Set for Children with Chronic Conditions*, July 3, 2008. As of October 22, 2020:
https://www.ahrq.gov/sites/default/files/wysiwyg/cahps/surveys-guidance/item-sets/children-chronic/102_Children_with_Chronic_Conditions_Set_2008.pdf

———, "About CAHPS," webpage, March 2020. As of October 22, 2020:
https://www.ahrq.gov/cahps/about-cahps

Althouse, Andrew D., "Adjust for Multiple Comparisons? It's Not That Simple," *Annals of Thoracic Surgery*, Vol. 101, No. 5, 2016, pp. 1644–1645.

Aronson, Keith R., Sandee J. Kyler, Jeremy D. Moeller, and Daniel F. Perkins, "Understanding Military Families Who Have Dependents with Special Health Care and/or Educational Needs," *Disability and Health Journal*, Vol. 9, No. 3, July 2016, pp. 423–430.

Backhus, Stephen P., Director, Veterans' Affairs and Military Health Care Issues, U.S. General Accounting Office, "Military Health Care: TRICARE's Civilian Provider Networks," memo to Committee on Armed Forces, Subcommittee on Military Personnel, U.S. House of Representatives, Washington, D.C., GAO/HEHS-00-64R, March 13, 2000.

Berry, Jay G., Matt Hall, Eyal Cohen, Margaret O'Neill, and Chris Feudtner, "Ways to Identify Children with Medical Complexity and the Importance of Why," *Journal of Pediatrics*, Vol. 167, No. 2, May 2015, pp. 229–237.

Bethell, Christina D., Stephen J. Blumberg, Ruth E. Stein, Bonnie Strickland, Julie Robertson, and Paul W. Newacheck, "Taking Stock of the CSHCN Screener: A Review of Common Questions and Current Reflections," *Academic Pediatrics*, Vol. 15, No. 2, March–April 2015, pp. 165–176.

Blue Star Families, "Additional Survey Results," webpage, undated. As of October 22, 2020:
https://bluestarfam.org/survey-more-results

———, *Military Family Lifestyle Survey: Comprehensive Report*, Encinitas, Calif., 2018.

———, "Policy Priorities," factsheet, 2020. As of October 22, 2020:
https://bluestarfam.org/wp-content/uploads/2020/07/BSF-Policy-Priorities_200714.pdf

Brown, Ryan Andrew, Grant N. Marshall, Joshua Breslau, Coreen Farris, Karen Chan Osilla, Harold Alan Pincus, Teague Ruder, Phoenix Voorhies, Dionne Barnes-Proby, Katherine Pfrommer, Lisa Kraus, Yashodhara Rana, and David M. Adamson, "Access to Behavioral Health Care for Geographically Remote Service Members and Dependents in the U.S.," *RAND Health Quarterly*, Vol. 5, No. 1, 2015. As of October 22, 2020:
https://www.rand.org/pubs/periodicals/health-quarterly/issues/v5/n1/21.html

Busacker, Ashley, and Laurin Kasehagen, "Association of Residential Mobility with Child Health: An Analysis of the 2007 National Survey of Children's Health," *Maternal and Child Health Journal*, Vol. 16, Suppl. 1, April 2012, pp. S78–S87.

CFR—*See* Code of Federal Regulations.

Children's Hospital Association, "Pediatric Specialist Physician Shortages Affect Access to Care," Washington, D.C., August 2012. As of October 22, 2020:
https://www.childrenshospitals.org/-/media/Files/CHA/Main/Issues_and_Advocacy/Key_Issues/Graduate_Medical_Education/Fact_Sheets/Pediatric_Specialist_Physician_Shortages_Affect_Access_to_Care08012012.pdf

Code of Federal Regulations, Title 32, National Defense, Section 199.17, TRICARE Program, current as of October 20, 2020.

Defense Health Agency, *Evaluation of the TRICARE Program: Fiscal Year 2017 Report to Congress*, Washington, D.C.: U.S. Department of Defense, June 8, 2017.

———, *Evaluation of the TRICARE Program: Fiscal Year 2019 Report to Congress*, Washington, D.C.: U.S. Department of Defense, July 9, 2019.

———, *Evaluation of the TRICARE Program: Fiscal Year 2020 Report to Congress*, Washington, D.C.: U.S. Department of Defense, June 29, 2020.

Defense Health Board, *Pediatric Health Care Services*, Falls Church, Va.: Office of the Assistant Secretary of Defense for Health Affairs, December 18, 2017.

DHA—*See* Defense Health Agency.

DHB—*See* Defense Health Board.

DoD—*See* U.S. Department of Defense.

Donovan, Fred, "DHA Lays Out 4 Objectives for Medical Treatment Facilities Transfer," *HIT Infrastructure*, August 27, 2019. As of October 22, 2020: https://hitinfrastructure.com/news/dha-lays-out-4-objectives-for-medical-treatment-facilities-transfer

Feise, Ronald J., "Do Multiple Outcome Measures Require p-Value Adjustment?" *BMC Medical Research Methodology*, Vol. 2, June 17, 2002, article 8.

Fowler, M. G., G. A. Simpson, and K. C. Schoendorf, "Families on the Move and Children's Health Care," *Pediatrics*, Vol. 91, No. 5, May 1993, pp. 934–940.

GAO—*See* U.S. Government Accountability Office.

Gleason, Jessica L., and Kenneth H. Beck, "Examining Associations Between Relocation, Continuity of Care, and Patient Satisfaction in Military Spouses," *Military Medicine*, Vol. 182, Nos. 5–6, 2017, pp. e1657–e1664.

Hero, Joachim O., Robert J. Blendon, Alan M. Zaslavsky, and Andrea L. Campbell, "Understanding What Makes Americans Dissatisfied with Their Health Care System: An International Comparison," *Health Affairs*, Vol. 35, No. 3, March 2016, pp. 502–509.

Institute for Healthcare Improvement, "IHI Triple Aim Initiative," webpage, undated. As of October 20, 2020: http://www.ihi.org/Engage/Initiatives/TripleAim/Pages/default.aspx

Jelleyman, T., and N. Spencer, "Residential Mobility in Childhood and Health Outcomes: A Systematic Review," *Journal of Epidemiology and Community Health*, Vol. 62, No. 7, July 2008, pp. 584–592.

Kanof, Marjorie, Director, Health Care—Clinical and Military Health Care Issues, U.S. General Accounting Office, *Defense Health Care: Oversight of the Adequacy of TRICARE's Civilian Provider Network Has Weaknesses*, testimony before the Committee on Armed Services, Subcommittee on Total Force, U.S. House of Representatives, Washington, D.C., GAO-03-592T, March 27, 2003.

Kerr, Eve A., Ron D. Hays, Allison Mitchinson, Martin Lee, and Albert L. Siu, "The Influence of Gatekeeping and Utilization Review on Patient Satisfaction," *Journal of General Internal Medicine*, Vol. 14, No. 5, May 1999, pp. 287–296.

Kongstvedt, Peter R., *Essentials of Managed Health Care*, Burlington, Mass.: Jones and Bartlett Learning, 2013.

Lichstein, Jesse C., Reem M. Ghandour, and Marie Y. Mann, "Access to the Medical Home Among Children with and Without Special Health Care Needs," *Pediatrics*, Vol. 142, No. 6, December 2018, article e20181795.

Mathematica Policy Research, *2010 Health Care Survey of DoD Beneficiaries: Child Technical Manual*, Washington, D.C., October 2010. As of October 22, 2020: https://tricare.mil/survey/hcsurvey/2009/ChildTechnicalManual_FY2009.pdf

Mayer, Michelle L., "Are We There Yet? Distance to Care and Relative Supply Among Pediatric Medical Subspecialties," *Pediatrics*, Vol. 118, No. 6, December 2006, pp. 2313–2321.

MHS—*See* Military Health System.

Military Health System, "MHS Facilities," online database, various dates. As of October 22, 2020:
https://www.health.mil/Military-Health-Topics/Access-Cost-Quality-and-Safety/
Patient-Portal-for-MHS-Quality-Patient-Safety-and-Access-Information/
See-How-Were-Doing/MTF-Results

———, *Section 709 of the National Defense Authorization Act for Fiscal Year 2017 (Public Law 114-328): Report on a Standardized System for Scheduling Medical Appointments at Military Treatment Facilities*, Washington, D.C.: U.S. Department of Defense, 2017.

Military OneSource, "The Exceptional Family Member Program: A Program for Families with Special Needs," June 8, 2020. As of October 22, 2020:
https://www.militaryonesource.mil/family-relationships/
special-needs/exceptional-family-member/
the-exceptional-family-member-program-for-families-with-special-needs

National Institutes of Health, *Military-Connected Children with Special Health Care Needs and Their Families: Conference Summary and Recommendations*, Bethesda, Md., April 2014. As of October 22, 2020:
https://www.nichd.nih.gov/sites/default/files/about/meetings/2014/Documents/
military_families_summary.pdf

Newacheck, Paul W., Margaret McManus, Harriette B. Fox, Yun-Yi Hung, and Neal Halfon, "Access to Health Care for Children with Special Health Care Needs," *Pediatrics*, Vol. 105, No. 4, April 2000, pp. 760–766.

Office of the Secretary of Defense, *Report to Congressional Defense Committees: Study on Health Care and Related Support for Children of Members of the Armed Forces*, Washington, D.C.: U.S. Department of Defense, July 2014.

Paley, Blair, Patricia Lester, and Catherine Mogil, "Family Systems and Ecological Perspectives on the Impact of Deployment on Military Families," *Clinical Child and Family Psychology Review*, Vol. 16, No. 3, September 2013, pp. 245–265.

Penchansky, Roy, and J. William Thomas, "The Concept of Access: Definition and Relationship to Consumer Satisfaction," *Medical Care*, Vol. 19, No. 2, February 1981, pp. 127–140.

Perneger, Thomas V., "What's Wrong with Bonferroni Adjustments," *British Medical Journal*, Vol. 316, No. 7139, April 18, 1998, pp. 1236–1238.

Public Law 112-239, *National Defense Authorization Act for Fiscal Year 2013*, January 2, 2013.

Public Law 115-91, *National Defense Authorization Act for Fiscal Year 2018*, December 12, 2017.

Rothman, Kenneth T., "No Adjustments Are Needed for Multiple Comparisons," *Epidemiology*, Vol. 1, No. 1, January 1990, pp. 43–46.

Seshadri, Roopa, Douglas Strane, Meredith Matone, Karen Ruedisueli, and David M. Rubin, "Families with TRICARE Report Lower Health Care Quality and Access Compared to Other Insured and Uninsured Families," *Health Affairs*, Vol. 38, No. 8, August 2019, pp. 1377–1385.

So, Marvin, Russell F. McCord, and Jennifer W. Kaminski, "Policy Levers to Promote Access to and Utilization of Children's Mental Health Services: A Systematic Review," *Administration and Policy in Mental Health and Mental Health Services Research*, Vol. 46, No. 3, May 2019, pp. 334–351.

TRICARE, "Health Care Survey of DoD Beneficiaries: Child Survey 2010," 2009. As of October 22, 2020:
https://tricare.mil/survey/hcsurvey/2009/Child_Questionnaire_Q3FY10.pdf

———, "Covered Services: Case Management," webpage, last updated September 3, 2019. As of October 22, 2020:
https://tricare.mil/CoveredServices/SpecialNeeds/CaseManagement.aspx

U.S. Census Bureau, "National Survey of Children's Health (NSCH)," webpage, undated. As of October 22, 2020:
https://www.census.gov/programs-surveys/nsch.html

U.S. Department of Defense, *2018 Demographics: Profile of the Military Community*, Washington, D.C., 2018a.

———, *Report to the Armed Services Committees: The Plan to Improve Pediatric Care for Children of Members of the Armed Forces*, Washington, D.C., December 2018b.

U.S. Department of Defense, TRICARE Management Activity, *Report on the Efficacy and Cost of Case Management Services for TRICARE Behavioral Health Clients with Serious Mental Health Problems*, Washington, D.C., April 2013.

U.S. General Accounting Office, *Military Personnel: Longer Time Between Moves Related to Higher Satisfaction and Retention*, Washington, D.C., GAO-01-841, August 2001.

U.S. Government Accountability Office, *Military Personnel: DoD Should Improve Its Oversight of the Exceptional Family Member Program*, Washington D.C., GAO-18-348, May 8, 2018.

———, *DoD Health Care: Improvements Needed for Tracking Coordination of Specialty Care Referrals for TRICARE Prime Beneficiaries*, Washington, D.C., GAO-19-488, June 2019.

Williams, Thomas V., Eric M. Schone, Nancy D. Archibald, and Joseph W. Thompson, "A National Assessment of Children with Special Health Care Needs: Prevalence of Special Needs and Use of Health Care Services Among Children in the Military Health System," *Pediatrics*, Vol. 114, No. 2, August 2004, pp. 384–393.

Wong, Charlene A., Kristin Kan, Zuleyha Cidav, Robert Nathenson, and Daniel Polsky, "Pediatric and Adult Physician Networks in Affordable Care Act Marketplace Plans," *Pediatrics*, Vol. 139, No. 4, April 2017, article e201631117.